How to Bicycle Across America

SHANE HANNAN

PAGE PUBLISHING, INC.
New York, NY

First originally published by Page Publishing, Inc. 2018

Cover Picture: May 2013 – Finishing at the famous Alamo in San Antonio, Texas.
Back Cover Picture: May 2011 – Somewhere between Glamis and Palo Verde, California.

ISBN 978-1-64214-929-6 (Paperback)
ISBN 978-1-64214-930-2 (Digital)

Printed in the United States of America

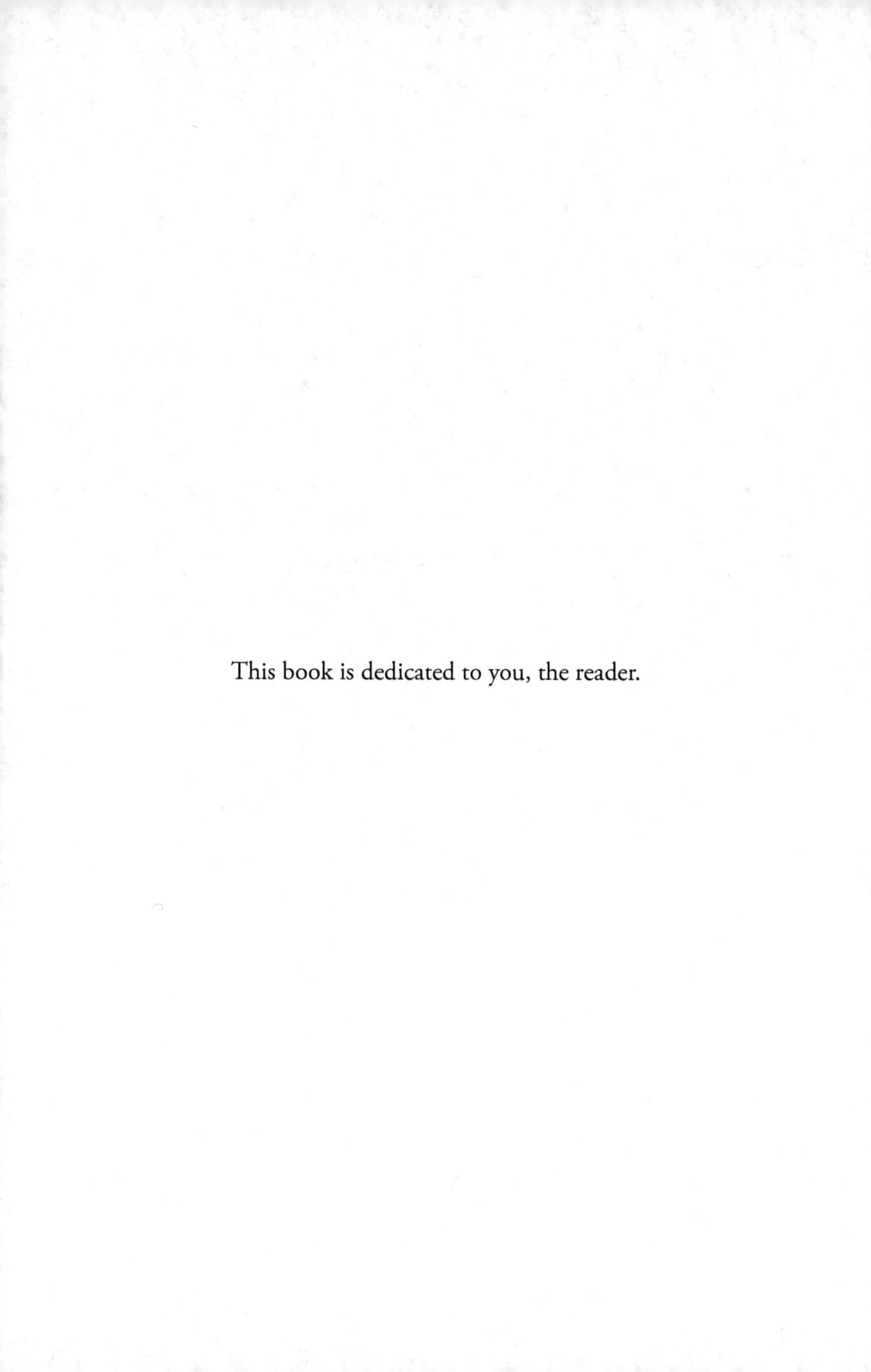

This book is dedicated to you, the reader.

CONTENTS

HOW TO BICYCLE ACROSS AMERICA

San Diego, California to San Augustine, Florida – distance 2,820 miles. 4,541 kilometers.

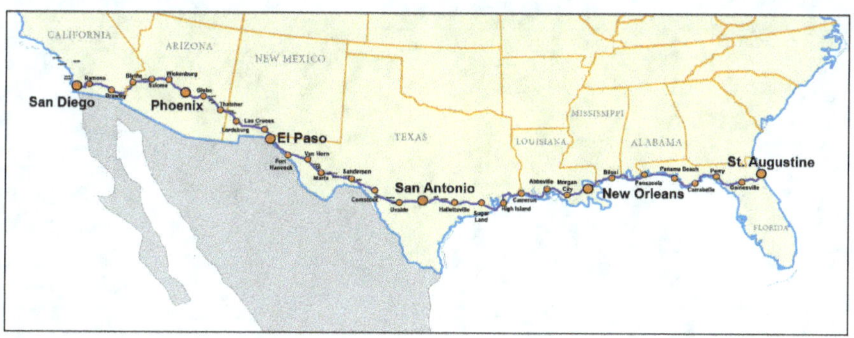

1.   San Diego to Phoenix – May 5–10, 2011 – 437 miles/703 kilometers – 6 days
2.   Phoenix to El Paso – May 30–June 4, 2012 – 430 miles/692 kilometers – 5 days
3.   El Paso to San Antonio – May 2–8, 2013 – 619 miles/966 kilometers – 7 days
4.   San Antonio to New Orleans – September 20–26, 2014 – 653 miles/1,051 kilometers – 7 days
5.   New Orleans to St. Augustine – November 1–7, 2015 – 681 miles/1,096 kilometers – 7 days

CHAPTER 1

This and That

We all have a bike story, right? Maybe the first time you rode a bike. At some point in your life you had a bike, were given a bike, borrowed a bike, or thought about buying a bike.

Once you learned how to ride, the bike was freedom. The thrill of speed going down a hill back then still generates the same feeling today. Rolling down a hill on a bike is timeless; you are no specific age when the wind is in your face and your motion is forward and effortless.

My first bicycle had no gears and had only a back pedal brake. It was a Matchless, which is one of the oldest marques of British motorcycles, manufactured in Plumstead, London, between 1899 and 1966. They built bicycles as well. After all, bicycles were around before motorbikes. I remember as a youngster going to the bike shop with my grandfather to buy that bike. It was a secondhand bike, but the frame was completely repainted in blue and red with all the fancy white pin striping and the wheel rims were hand-painted in blue and white to match.

I spent hours sitting on the saddle with feet on the pedals, holding onto a nearby post or fence because I didn't know how to ride. We would go to the park and grandfather would give me a big push and away I'd go. I can still feel the acceleration of the start! This was enough to gain the confidence of balance. Of course, the next problem was stopping, which usually ended with me on the grass with a skinned knee.

I'd ride for what seemed like hours around that park. Didn't take long before that push start wasn't needed and I was free to ride whenever. Grandfather must have gotten a real thrill out of watching my sister and me learning how to ride our bikes. I remember my kids, learning to ride, and what an accomplishment I thought it was for them.

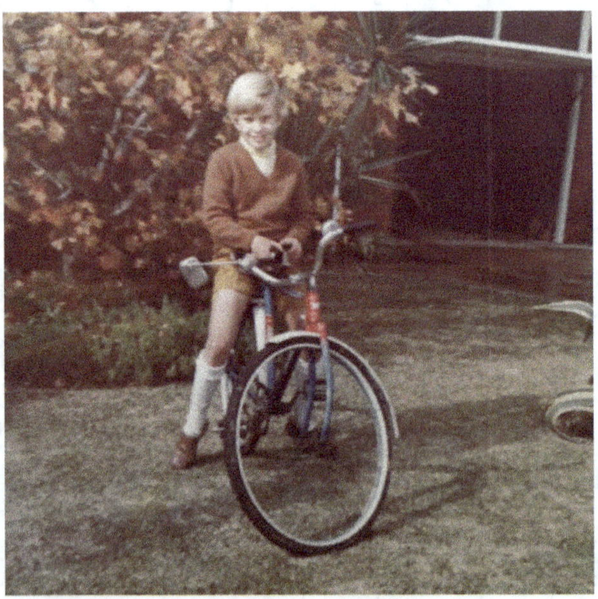

Yep. That's me on my Matchless bicycle.

Why Such a Ride?

Bicycling has been a solid friend over the years. It's given me the opportunity to get away from everything, let my brain wonder, solve problems, and get a little exercise.

Weekend rides around the beaches of the Sutherland Shire and through the Royal National Park were always a weekend treat. I would usually do this with my Aussie mate, Darryl, who was partly the inspiration for my ride (see *My Mid-Life Crisis* by Darryl Chappelow). I can remember us riding one sunny morning on a lonely road through the Nasho (Royal National Park) and discussing the possibility of bicycling around Australia, how long it would take, and what a great adventure that would be. Not more than ten minutes later, two cyclists came along in the opposite direction fully loaded with gear. As they passed, we asked their destination, and in a European accent, they replied, "We are viding around Os'tralia."

My dad said to me one time, "Don't miss the opportunity to do something now, because when you get older, you will wish you had."

At the time, I'd lived in the States for fifteen years, traveling all over the US, spending a lot of time on airplanes or in rental cars. The airplane window is a moving picture of the world below with different terrains, big and small cities, deserts, mountains, rivers and roads. You know what, I'd think to myself, I could probably ride across that.

Maybe all this was just building up for riding coast to coast across America. Morning meetings at the coffee shop only added more fuel to the idea. There were a couple of other blokes who also showed interest in riding across America. Our discussions continued until about two weeks before the deadline to buy the airline ticket to San Diego. At this point, I made the decision to go it alone.

Timing and Planning

It seemed like the timing was right. The kids were really growing up, with Kate in high school and Jake starting college. I'd been back to visit my family in Australia every couple of years. Business was recovering from the 2009 recession. My wife, Sara, was willing to tolerate my idea about riding across the US. My fiftieth birthday was fast approaching. It was time to do *something!* Something big!

I started planning my potential ride, but really couldn't take a month or longer away from my business. (It's a bloody long way mate!) But Darryl had the answer. Break the journey down into segments like he did, riding around Australia one month at a time over five years. Okay, that's easy – take a week and do a section each year, flying in and out of the start and finish points. It became an exciting personal project – putting everything together, looking at potential routes, studying different bike equipment, and of course, training. Besides, taking the journey in stages over five years would give me something else to look forward to – the detailed planning out of each stage of the ride.

What can go wrong? What's the worst that can happen? The positives continued to add up more than the negatives. I could get hit by a car or truck. Yes, that is true. There might be snakes, mountain lions, bears, and oh yeah, the crazy dogs, which I never really took into consideration. But I thought, "I can do this! After all it's only one week a year, cycling from one destination to the next. I'm not the first person to do this. I'm sure people do this all the time!" And sure enough, they do – quite a lot of interesting characters, some solo, some in groups, and some in an organized and fully supported trip.

There are a number of different routes a bicyclist can take. Some go San Diego to New York. Others like Seattle to New York or Seattle to Miami – each with various challenges. The most logical was the southern route starting in San Diego, taking me back through Phoenix and the southern states. (And besides, I don't really like the cold weather.) There are plenty of blogs on the Internet about people traveling on bicycles all over the United States and the world. These were a great help for planning and what to expect on the road. This was a great site: https://www.crazyguyonabike.com/.

Next was to break each section of the ride down into six or seven days, then focusing on that one stage of the ride until it was completed. I would spend hours on the weekend reading other cyclist's blogs on the Internet and their experiences riding across America.

Planning out each day of a stage was a lot of fun: how far apart are the hotels, food stops, water needs, the terrain (hill vs. flat), the seasonal wind direction, and overall weather conditions. Google Maps/Earth were great for zooming in and seeing road conditions, width of road shoulder, and roadside facilities along the way. Scrolling along roads with my mouse was a virtual preride. The mapping was also excellent for calculating the distance and time needed between stops.

My Bike

For a ride like this you need a bike that is reliable – one that you know how to do basic repairs on in case you break down on a back road. On certain parts of the route, there's not a lot of traffic, especially on some of the roads. It may take quite a while for someone to come by to help, *if* they stop, or you have a long walk to civilization.

You don't necessarily need an expensive bike to do this type of ride. I found along the way that people would be riding all types of bikes, from high-end to something that looked like they found it on the side of the road. It really comes down to what is comfortable for you.

My bike is a Navaro Divano from REI, made of aluminum with carbon fiber front forks. I purchased the bike on sale years ago for $650. Since then, the running gear has been replaced twice, along with brakes and many sets of tubes and tires.

The seat on my bike is stock seat and has proven very "reliable" over the years. People have suggested better quality brands, but if something is working, why change it?

Prior to each stage of the ride, I would have my bike fully serviced. It was part of the preparation and helped boost my confidence that mechanically everything on the bike would be okay for the trip. After a service, the bike always felt a lot smoother going through the gears, braking and handling.

I'd put on a new set of tires for each section of the trip, and the last three stages of the ride I used Continental Gatorskins tires. The first two stages of the ride I used Serfas tires with the FPS (flat protection strip). These were okay, but nothing like the Gatorskin tires. I've found the 25-mm wide tires the best fit for me (less drag than the 28-mm tires and wider than 23-mm tires for more comfort).

Equipment

I can't say enough about tribars. This additional equipment that clamps onto the existing handlebars gives you more riding positions, from sitting up to leaning low across the bike as needed. This also helps take the weight off your bum and distribute your weight along the bike. The tribars are great for attaching equipment like GPS, phone, extended mirror, front light, and a bell. I'd refer to this area as the cockpit. Everything needed during the day was right there.

I had a rack on the back to carry rear panniers. The Racktime panniers were great with lots of external pockets for various things and easily clipped on the racking system. They also had built-in rain covers that did a pretty good job, considering they endured a very rainy 10 hours in one day. I would put a safety strap across the top to tie the two together in case one might fall off. The clip-on / clip-off system on the panniers worked great, but I would ride for sometimes hours without looking back. I only used rear panniers for the ride. If you are planning on camping out, then you would also need front panniers for the extra gear.

For the first two stages of the ride, San Deigo–Phoenix–El Paso, I wore regular sporting shoes, Pumas. The bike came with toe clip pedals where you can pull the strap down to hold your foot in place. I never had the straps tight, just loose fitting in case I needed to get out in a hurry.

From El Paso on, I changed out the toe clip pedals for clip-ins, or SPD system (Shimano Pedaling Dynamics). This involves a small cleat which is fitted in the recess of the sole of a shoe, which then clips into the bike's pedal. They took a bit getting comfortable with, knowing that I was firmly attached to the bike. The first week with them on, I had a couple of incidents not getting out of the clips in time when stopping. The result was just falling sideways, which I'm sure provided a few laughs for anyone watching me. I have to tell you that once you do get used to them, they are great and very easy to use. I used the Shimano SLX M530 clipless pedals paired with Shimano MT33L shoes. These clipless pedals and shoes are more suited for mountain biking. I liked the shoes because the metal cleat is located up in the sole making it easier to walk around, so no need for an extra pair of shoes when packing. Other clip-in shoes have the metal cleat protruding from the sole and are tough to walk in.

I would carry two bottles of water attached to the bicycle frame, 22 ounces each, 44 ounces (1.3 liters) all in all, along with an additional 70 ounces (2 liters) of water in a CamelBak/backpack. As long as you are careful, this would last between water stops. I'd usually grab a large bottle of Gatorade and consume that during the day as well. It's really important to keep hydrated when doing long rides. After riding a while, your body will let you know when to drink and when to eat.

I tried out a number of different types of rear-vision mirrors prior to starting the trip. The ones that clip on the helmet were super small and I needed to adjust my head every time to see behind. I ended up with a cycling mirror that was fairly large, mounted on the side of my tribars. Sure, it looks a little awkward sticking out past the handlebars, but it was perfect to see any potential danger coming from behind and hopefully provide enough time to get out of the way. The large mirror was also something else to monitor or help to entertain me on those long days, looking down to check traffic behind, plus it gave me a bit more peace of mind.

My standard equipment list is as follows:

- One bike lock – for the rare times my bike would be out of my vision.
- A compact set of bike tools that includes a tool to fix a broken chain.
- Twelve tire repair patches, as they come in packs of six. You never know, right?
- Three spare tubes, which were just enough at one point in New Mexico on the Interstate 10 Highway.
- One fold-up spare tire.
- A compact hand pump.
- One big knife . . . It's an Aussie thing.
- Pepper spray, just in case.

On my first stage of the ride, I travelled with too much stuff. As each stage progressed, I would carry less, especially once across west Texas and back in "civilization" where towns and cities are not as far away from each other. It would be easy to just buy anything extra I needed from a local store. I also got into a system of packing, so I knew where to go for food, tools, puncture kits, spare tire, and various clothing. Everything was stored in the same place for easy and quick access.

As far as what to take regarding clothing, it depends on the time of year and the climate. Less weight is always best when going up a hill or spending the day against a headwind. But you still need to consider having enough food, water, and clothing. Don't try crossing the deserts in summer or the mountain ranges in winter, although a lot of people have. I prefer a mild climate and sunny weather where I can travel with less gear. Some areas have limited or no amenities for food or accommodations, so planning out your route is essential in determining how much water and food you need to carry. Once across the desert states, there are more places and choices for food and accommodations, so your luggage and amount of supplies needed can be a lot less. The lighter the load to carry, the better!

Other equipment is a phone and maybe a GPS. I started with a Garmin GPS, but as the technology got better with maps and phones, I relied more on the phone. It was amazing how quickly the technology changed from GPS maps to apps like www.mapmyride.com that track the entire ride. There was a significant difference in my daily reports over the 5 years that showed better maps that included elevation, speed, and calories burned. Due to copyright laws on certain maps, the book has generic maps. For more detailed maps, visit – www.howtobicycleacrossamerica.com

The other aspect of maps is planning the best route for a trip like this, and sometimes the complexity of navigating through a big city. Once clear of the city you are generally limited to one or two different roads, so navigating isn't that difficult.

Each day would start out fairly early on the road in the dark. It was really important to have good lighting so the predawn drivers were able to clearly see me. Some of the road shoulders weren't that generous, so at times I would be traveling close to speeding vehicles. I even had lights on my helmet.

To keep the phone at maximum level throughout the day, I would plug into an external battery pack when starting out, which worked really well. When I arrived at a hotel, the first job would be to take a shower/bath, and second was to get all the electronics charged up for the next day.

I also found an app that I could use on my phone that would track my exact location on a map – www.greenalp.com. This was great for people who wanted to track my progress live and know exactly where I was on the road.

Some people do this ride and camp out every night along the way. I really take my hat off to those people. When camping out, they carry a lot more gear than I would. More gear means more weight. Also, the added complexity of finding a suitable and safe campsite each evening and pitching a tent versus booking a reasonable hotel online, then arriving to a comfortable bed, hot shower, and cooked breakfast (sometimes anyway) – this was an easy choice for me.

Training

Already I was riding about 3,000 miles (4,828 kilometers) a year or 60 miles (97 kilometers) a week around Phoenix. I hadn't completed a long day ride, so I was determined to complete at least 100 miles (160 kilometers) in one day. I thought this would be the magic number to ensure I could make the distance between hotels or food and water in some parts of the cross-country ride. I built up to this distance over a period of time, starting out riding at least three times a week, averaging 20 miles (32 kilometers) each ride. I built up the miles from there to an average of 115 miles (185 kilometers) per week. Once I completed my first "century" ride, I was confident I could make it between facilities, unless I had a problem with the bike that I couldn't fix. Then I'd just have to thumb a lift or walk.

The human body is really an amazing thing. I was surprised at how well my body responded to such a big change in mileage day after day once I started each stage. Going from 115 miles (185 kilometers) in a week to almost 700 miles (1,100 kilometers) was a big change.

My average day was about 90 miles (141 kilometers) distance and average speed of 15 miles (24 kilometers) an hour, although the shortest day was 65 miles (105 kilometers) and the longest day 126 miles (202 kilometers). This all depended on the location of a town and accommodations each day. When mapping this out prior to the trip, I would try to go as far as possible each day.

The daily routine would also start out early, riding a few hours before breakfast, then I'd get back on and ride another three or four hours before lunch. This would leave the afternoon for maybe three or four hours, before ending the day and dinner.

There are some people who complete this adventure doing 25 to 45 miles (40 to 102 kilometers) a day. You don't have to be cycling 100 miles (160 kilometers) plus a day to do this. The journey will take longer, but you probably get to see and experience more of the sights along the way. You may have more spare time. I guess it all comes down to a person just wanting to do it. Just make sure you're prepared, ride the distance you can each day, and never ever give up!

Motivation

Traveling with my laptop was a must. The slight increase in weight wasn't that significant. It allowed me to keep on top of work stuff, check weather conditions, book hotels, etc. Each night, after cleaning up, I would do a small email about my day's adventure. These daily updates started out as a quick summary to my family and friends, letting them know I finished safely that day, where I was that evening, and any entertaining events that I'd come across. They became a highly enjoyable reading experience by most, to the point that if I missed sending the daily update I'd get a bunch of email or phone calls asking for it. These daily updates became the basis for this book.

The responses from people reading these turned into something that I never anticipated. They were as hungry for this adventure as I was. They wanted to fully experience it, even if it was just through reading my stories. This became a real motivation for me. Each day on the road, I would think about my friends reading these updates, my relationships with them, their lives and families, and their situations.

The daily updates almost became bigger than the ride itself, as I found myself taking more time each night to clearly explain my thoughts, the surroundings, the different smells I was experiencing, and interesting people I met along the way.

Onward

It was time to do this and I was ready, and the weather was right; it was late May. The mountain elevations of the Sierra Nevada's were not too cold and the heat of the Anza-Borrego Desert was bearable. Although a bunch of mates were aware of my pending adventure, I still didn't encourage any of them to join me. It was to be a solo adventure, which did cause a bit of concern – traveling alone, on a bike. Sometimes, as it turned out, being in the middle of nowhere and being alone became one of the best parts of the whole experience. The coming and going as I pleased, not having to worry about a travelling companion or their schedule. The time alone, deeply immersed in the adventure and meeting people along the way was a real treat.

Hopefully, you will enjoy the journey as much as I did!

CHAPTER 2

San Diego, California,
to Phoenix, Arizona
May 5–May 10, 2011

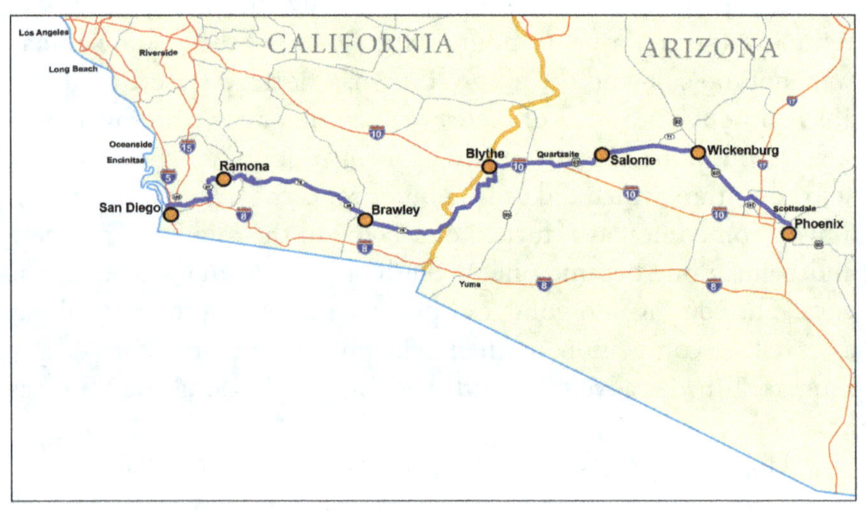

Total distance – 440 miles/708 kilometers
Number of days – 6
Average speed – 15 mph/24 kph
Total saddle time – 35 hours
Total climb – 10,289 ft/3,136 meters
Total descent – 9,242 ft/2,816 meters

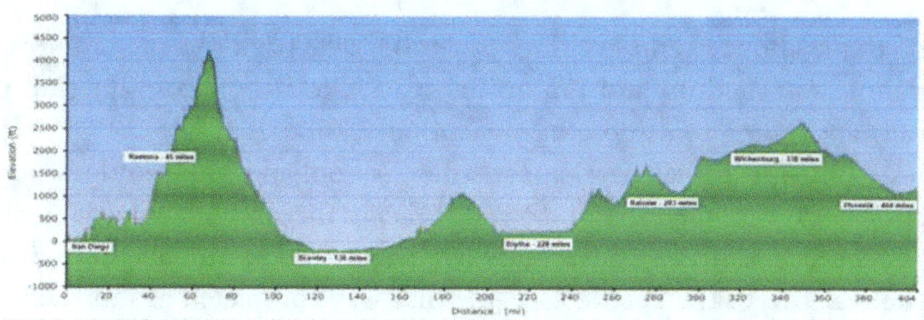

Elevation Change.

Day 1: Thursday, May 5, 2011

San Diego to Ramona, California – 47 miles/76 kilometers

Well, this is it! I'm excited and concerned at the same time, with many different thoughts going through my head as Sara drives me to the airport. It's the first flight at 6:00 a.m. from Phoenix to San Diego for the start of the ride. I'm sure she has similar thoughts . . . Is this the last time I see him? Did I pay his life insurance this month? She has since told me she was less worried about me traveling back roads in unknown places than riding around Scottsdale with the morning traffic.

At the curb, I unload my boxed bike with one small carryon bag. She gives me a kiss and wishes me good luck. I drag my boxed bike into the terminal. I'm on my own now.

Looking out the plane window of this fifty-minute flight I see the roads, mountains and deserts, I will be going over and traveling through. Fifty minutes on a plane is the equivalent of approximately five days on a bicycle covering the same distance.

The plane lands right on time at 8:05 a.m. Pacific Standard Time. My bike doesn't turn up on the baggage carousel; the box is oversized. My bike arrives at a separate door. It's a busy morning in baggage claim with people dressed in business attire or beach gear waiting for their luggage. My presence in bike shorts and a green fluoro top, unpacking my bike and gear, helps them to pass the time. It takes me about twenty minutes to get the bike back together and my panniers packed up and I'm on my way. The airport baggage claim staff are willing to dispose of my cardboard bike box.

Outside the airport the weather is cool, no wind and sunny skies, with the smell of salt from the Pacific Ocean. I'm heading west to Ocean Beach as it's customary for a coast-to-coast bike trip to dip the rear tire in the Pacific Ocean. That was completed around 9:30 a.m. From there I biked to a friend's location in Mission Valley to stock up on water and pick up my bike glasses, which were shipped there from the eyewear company.

Leaving Mission Valley at 10:30 a.m. was the start of navigating out of the city with my state-of-the-art BlackBerry Torch mobile phone while watching for traffic. The nice thing about this mapping app on the phone is that it gives alternate routes and includes highlighted bicycle ways.

I'm now at Mission Trails Regional Park, which is the start of a 15-mile walking/bike trail. As I come through the park entry, I attract the attention of the park caretakers, Ed and his wife, Ruth. Ed is a retired San Diego County sheriff who was born in Julian, the town I will be going through tomorrow at the top of the Sierra Mountains. Ed tells me he used to ride up that hill when he was a young bloke and provides guidance on the road ahead. They are both suddenly distracted by a busload of visitors, so I ride on.

It's about noon and time for lunch at a Circle K on Highway 67 near Eucalyptus Hills. It felt like I'd been climbing hills since leaving the beach, but at this point I'm only 400 feet above sea level! A little depressing knowing I have 4,000 feet of uphill ahead of me.

The climb to Ramona is slow and hot – like 102° F at 5 to 9 miles per hour with plenty of traffic passing me. Halfway through this hill, it's time for a break in the shade. I hadn't gotten off the bike yet, but I noticed a large rattlesnake sliding along next to me heading for my intended shady tree. This might be a good photo opportunity . . . to hell with that, keep going. Cresting at 2,100 feet, I'm just outside Ramona, then an enjoyable few downhill miles into town.

I grabbed the only hotel in town and cleaned up. Good tip for bicycling and hotels: take the room on the ground floor so you don't have to lug your bike up the stairs. The hotel has no elevator so it was another climb to get to my room.

I'm not carrying too much weight; I was trying to keep everything to a minimum, but the cold weather gear I had packed probably won't be needed from here on in. So I head over to the post office and mail that gear home.

Tonight I celebrate my first day of riding with a grande Mexican feast and a few well deserved Coronas. Happy Cinco de Mayo! For a solo ride, I met lots of interesting and helpful people today.

Stats for the Day:

Distance – 47 miles/76 kilometers
Riding time – 4 hours 15 minutes
Average speed – 11.7 mph/18.8 kph
Elevation – 2,100 ft

The Route:

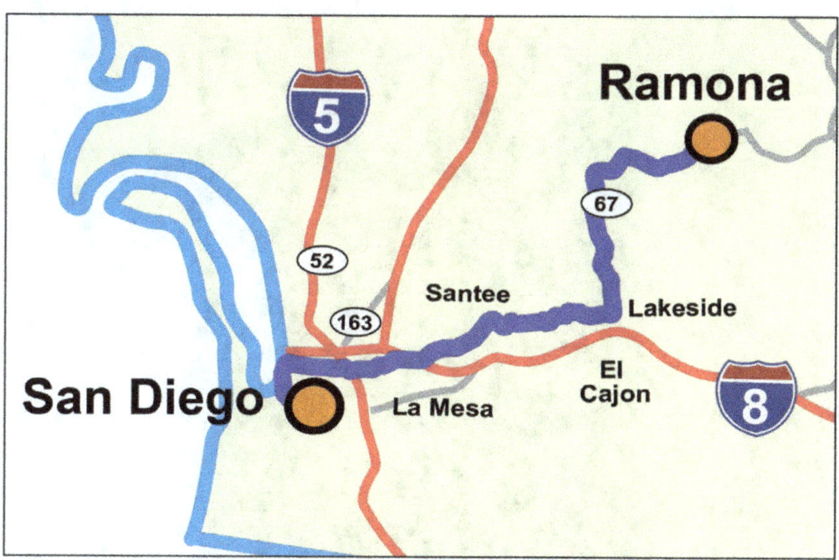

From San Diego Airport to Pacific Beach then east to Ramona, California.

Pictures of the Day:

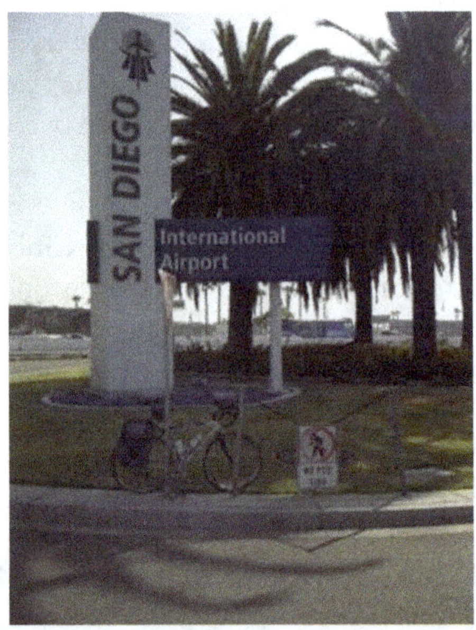

Leaving San Diego International Airport.

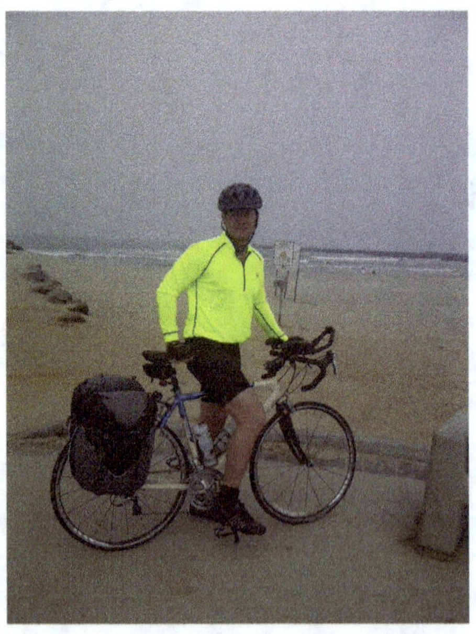

The official start Pacific Ocean at Ocean Beach, San Diego, California.

Day 2: Friday, May 6, 2011

Ramona to Brawley, California – 95 miles/153 kilometers

I thought roosters crowed at daybreak! Someone must have been shining a torch at the little guy, and he thought the sun was coming up at 2:30 a.m. Anyhow, I started out today at 5:30 a.m. in the dark and it's a cold 42°F degrees. After a 21-mile climb to 4,300 feet through some beautiful country, I arrived at the top of the mountain in Julian, California, at 8:00 a.m. It's a small town nestled in the Cuyamaca Mountains. I find a small coffee shop and the perfect time for a well-deserved breakfast.

The morning aches and pains of cycling uphill give way to a 10-mile downhill run with speeds at 30–40 mph. With the weight of my luggage, I keep having to slow the bike down. It would be no good to come off or blow a tire at this point!

The green countryside and tall trees soon give way to high desert views. Not much longer to the sandy remote Anza Borrego Desert along Highway 78. The geology and rock formations are alien like and there's hardly any traffic on this road.

Around 11:00 a.m. I come across a welcome rest stop in the desert called the Blu-In Café in Ocotillo Wells. It's just me and the cook, as the duners' (dirt bikes, four-wheelers, and RVs) season is over and the area is like a ghost town. The Blu-In Cafe is akin to something out of a Clint Eastwood movie, where he rides in on a horse and the bar door creaks as it's opened.

Besides a lot of sunscreen on my exposed skin, I tried out a wide brimmed hat today for extra protection. As soon as my speed exceeded 15 mph, the front of the brim would either go up, exposing my face to the sun, or go down covering my eyes, an unexpected failure. Back to my bike helmet . . .

The undulating desert landscape continues for about 20 miles till about 1:00 p.m. when I make a turn south onto Highway 86. Directly in front of me is the Salton Sea. This is an ancient sea that was landlocked from the Sea of Cortez in Mexico's Baja area many centuries ago. This area is lower than sea level and sometime in the 1800s was flooded by runoff from the Colorado River. These days, it's landlocked again and supports the irrigation for the farming in the area.

The afternoon sun is hot – 95°F in the shade and extra heat coming off the roadway. There's nothing out here to shelter under, unless you want to share a three foot high salt bush with a rattlesnake. Say no more, I ride on. But it's getting hotter and I need to take a break. I manage to get shelter from the sun in the shadow of a 65 mph signpost. I'm sweating, and my water is hot and running low. I look up and like a mirage in the desert, I see a small town up ahead – Westmoreland. At the gas station, I load up: Gatorade, ice cream, and a bag of chips.

It's about another eight miles into Brawley and tonight's hotel is the Best Western, which is not a bad place to stay. Even better, just across the road is the Imperial Chinese restaurant, so that will be dinner.

It was eight hours riding time today and over 90 miles closer to Phoenix. Five rest breaks to cool off and eat. I safely arrived in Brawley at 3:20 p.m.

Blythe, CA, tomorrow – 100 miles. Hope it's a little cooler!

Stats for the Day:

Distance – 95 miles/153 kilometers
Riding time – 8 hours
Average speed – 11.8 mph/19 kph
Elevation – 111 ft below sea level

The Route:

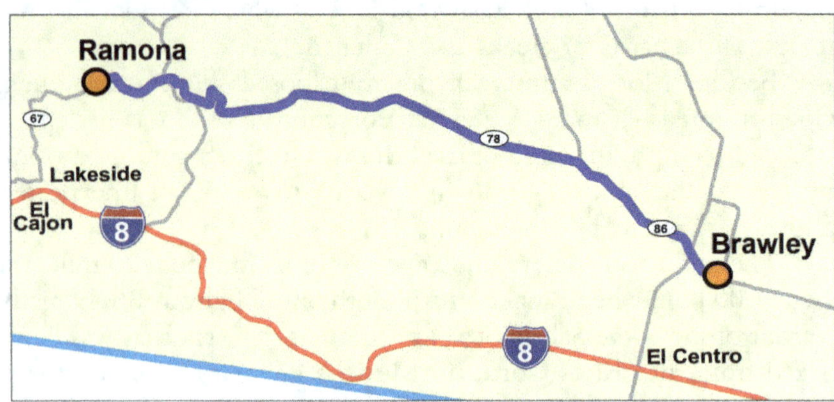

From Ramona to Brawley, California.

Pictures of the Day:

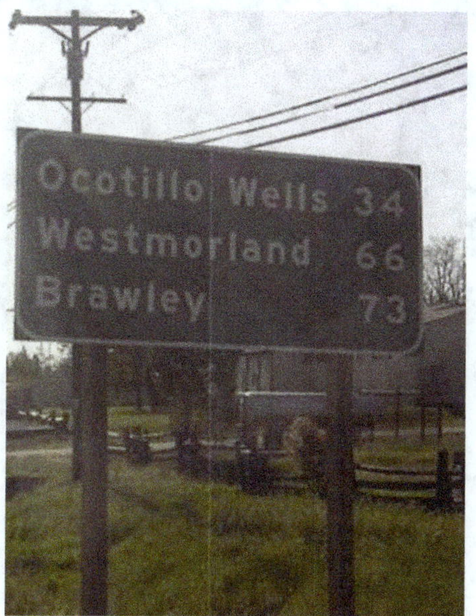

At the top of the mountains.

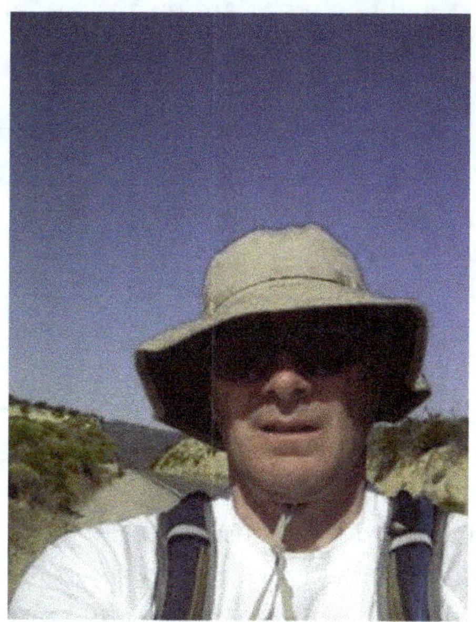

Floppy hat, all good until about 5 mph.

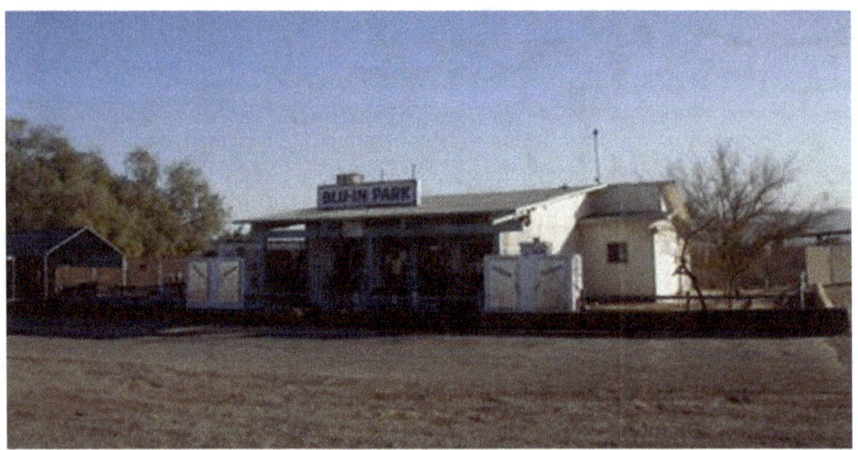

Blu-In Café, Ocotillo Wells, California.

Day 3: Saturday, May 7, 2011

Brawley to Blythe, California – 100 miles/161 kilometers

After a good night's sleep, I am on the road at 4:30 a.m. and cycling in the cool and dark. I can smell the water in the irrigation canal running alongside the road.

The green fields of Brawley are now behind me and the terrain turns to sandy desert. This area is known as the Imperial Sand Dunes, and this time of year is silent. In the winter months, it's a popular off road spot for four-wheel driving, dirt biking, and sand rails.

Enjoying the sight of another sunrise, I was surprised to see a person on a bicycle coming toward me. Who would be out here this time of day (or year)? I can just make out his outline with the sun shining directly at me. As I get closer, I hear, "G'day mate! Where you heading?" How funny, meeting another Aussie crossing the country on a bicycle. Richard has been on the road for eighty days starting in Saint Augustine, Florida, and is now only three days from completing his transcontinental crossing. Good job Richard! We have a good chat and exchange contact details. I ride on in amazement at another person on a bike in the middle of nowhere. I find out later that Richard has also sailed his boat from Florida to Australia.

I take a quick break at Glamis Beach store which is closed and deserted due to the end of the off-road / sand dune season. There's a nice tail wind developing from the west, and I'm now on Highway 78. Sixteen miles along, I come across a US border immigration checkpoint. They don't bother checking my credentials and I continue on.

This area is called the Chocolate Mountains (looks like chocolate cake, really). The area has some great scenery with the sandy desert running up the sides of the mountains, probably similar to the landscape on Mars!

At about 8:00 a.m. the wind is changing to a sow-westa (wind from the southwest), which is really helping to increase my speed. At some spots I'm cracking 22 mph. It's not long before I see another biker heading toward me. It's a girl riding with an organized group, making her way to Brawley against a strong headwind. I say "G'day," and through the passing traffic, we discuss road conditions, then eventually wish each other best of luck and a safe ride.

Another 40 miles and I make it to Palo Verde at 9:30 a.m. It's time for a break and a healthy food choice. So I settle for a well-deserved Klondyke bar – ice cream between two chocolate biscuits.

Palo Verde is part of Riverside County and the start of the agriculture area called the Lower Colorado River Valley. The road is on the west side of the river, and I follow this along through farms and irrigation canals on my way to Blythe.

The excellent tail wind seemed to blow me all the way along, and I arrive in Blythe at 11:30 a.m. The timing was perfect as the dry heat started to kick in. This was the longest day in miles that I needed to cover, and it is probably the most concerning because of the heat and such desolate areas between facilities. It turned out that leaving early this morning was a good decision!

Stats for the Day:

Distance – 100 miles/161 kilometers
Riding time – 7 hours
Average speed – 14.2 mph/22.8 kph
Elevation – 272 ft

The Route:

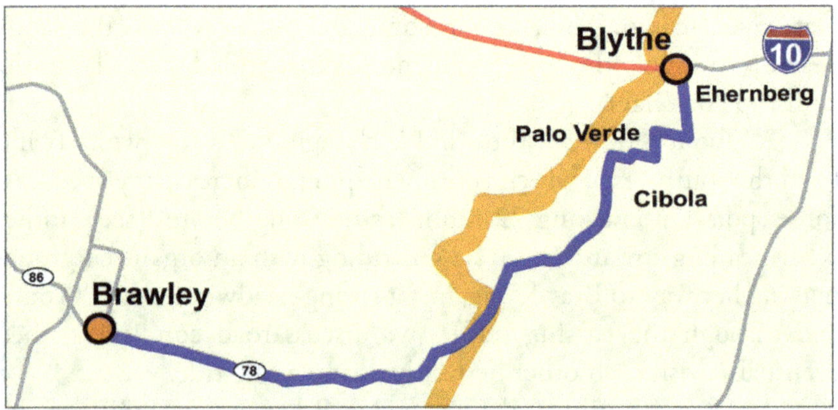

From Brawley to Blythe, California.

Pictures of the Day:

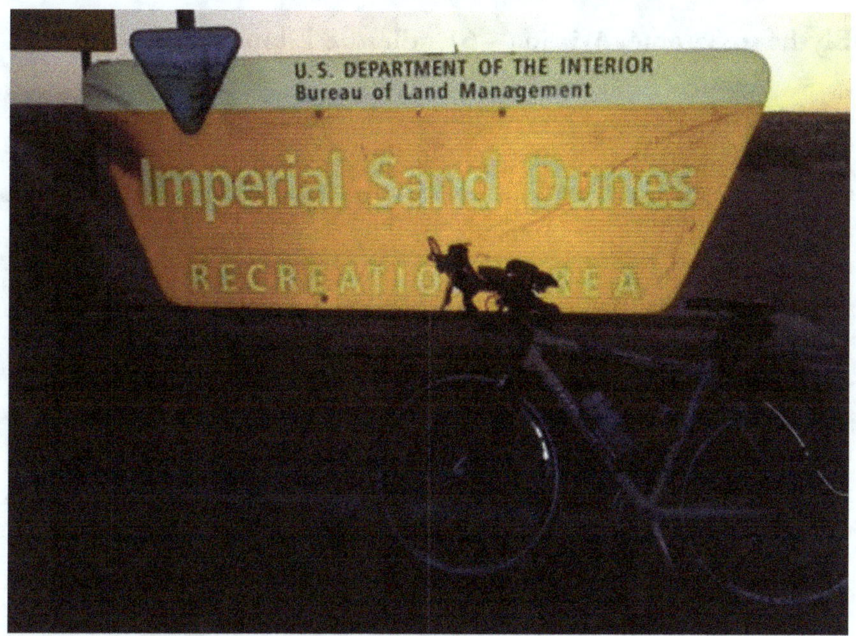

California Imperial Sand Dunes just before sunup.

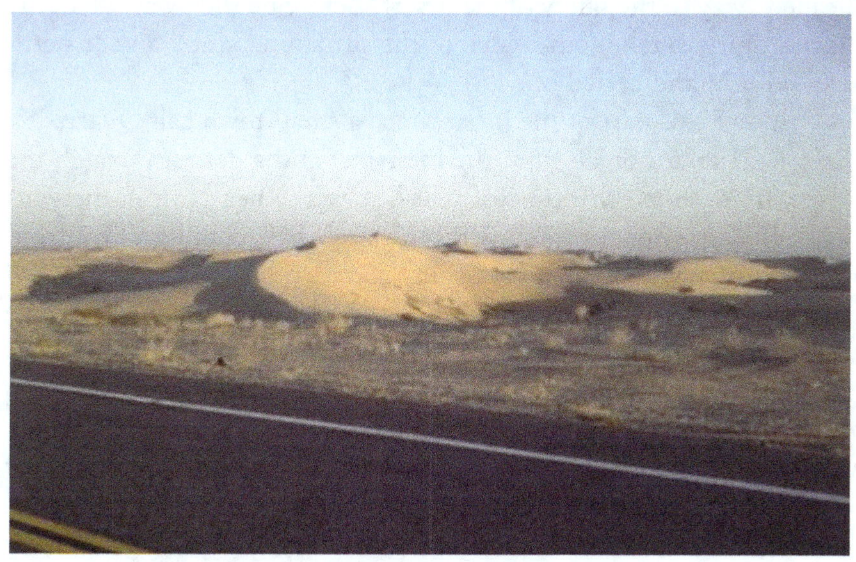

Sand dunes at sunrise.

Day 4: Sunday, May 8, 2011

Blythe to Salome, Arizona – 61 miles/98 kilometers

Happy Mother's Day, Mom!

On the road at 5:30 a.m. and soon I cross the Colorado River with Blythe behind me. I'm now in Arizona. Today's ride includes 35 miles riding on the Interstate 10 Highway. It's the first part of the ride, so I'm thinking there might be less traffic and less trucks as there are no other roads around this area. Riding on this is the only option. I did check with the Department of Public Safety (Highway Patrol), and the law states that if there is no alternative road, bicyclists can ride on the side of the interstate highways across the United States.

It's a big hill climbing out of the Blythe area, and on the last hill I encountered another rattlesnake, similarly sized to the snake on day one near Ramona, but this one is stretched across the shoulder. I only noticed it at the last minute as I had my head down, concentrating on getting up this hill. At this point I stop and start backing up. He was attempting to cross the interstate, but each passing truck made him coil up and in a pose, ready to strike! He eventually turned and headed away to the safety of the desert. Before he slid away, I had the opportunity to take some video of the situation. I took a wide berth around him and cycled on.

Along this part of the interstate is a small town call Quartzsite, Arizona. I take a break from the interstate and a detour through the town. It's deserted this time of year due to the heat, but in the winter, it fills up with snowboarders with their RVs coming down from the cold north. A large metal fishing rod catches my eye, along with a steering wheel from a boat and an anchor. This is the Quartzsite Yacht Club, but the riverbed is dry – no water, rivers, bays, or oceans for miles.

Although the shoulder lane on the interstate is wide, it still feels like the trucks are close as they speed by me. The speed and shape of the trucks generate a lot of wind in front and to the sides of them, causing a vacuum behind the truck. As they go by, I can feel my speed increasing as I cycle along.

I'm just ahead of an area called Dome Valley, and again the scenery is incredible with odd shaped mountains and hills all around me. From here, I can see for miles!

This is now the turn off for Highway US 60 and finally off of the interstate headed for Hope, Arizona. The roadway is very smooth and lonely, and the shoulder is generous enough and relaxing.

Fifteen miles out of Salome, I see another biker heading my way. This guy has been on the road for 77 days and looks pretty fit. He is pulling a one wheel trailer or a bob, and I see that he is eager to get to San Diego and be finished with his adventure. He is concerned about the route ahead and asks me a bunch of questions about the interstate and climbing through the mountains, then navigating through San Diego. I'm sure he will make it.

It's been a great day and I finished around noon in Salome, Arizona, at the Sheffler's Hotel. As I pull in I notice my front tire is squashy. My first flat tire and what a bonus; it's on the front wheel and just as I was pulling into the hotel.

I have a surprise guest tonight. Sara is meeting me for dinner and spending the night in Salome! We enjoy the activity and history at Don's Cactus Bar, a tour of the hotel shows where they used to hide slot machines between false walls back in the day.

Stats for the Day:

Distance – 61 miles/98 kilometers
Riding time – 5 hours 15 minutes
Average speed – 11.6 mph/18.7 kph
Elevation – 1,873 ft

The Route:

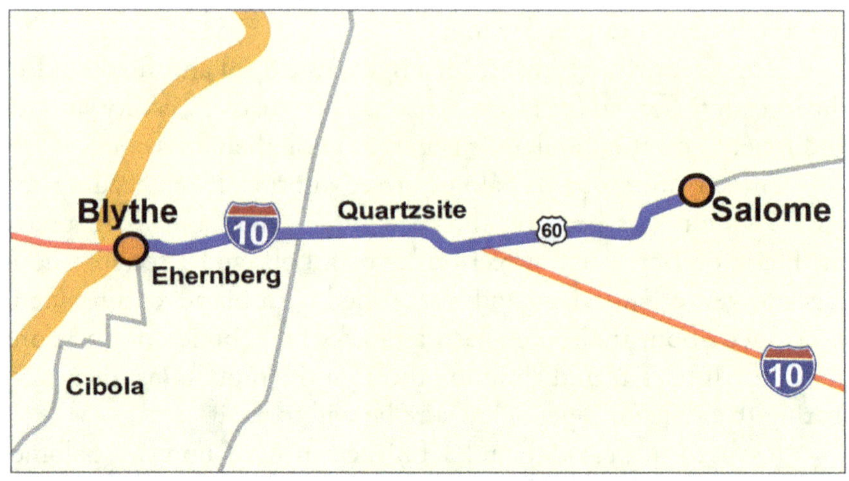

From Blythe, California, to Salome, Arizona.

Pictures of the Day:

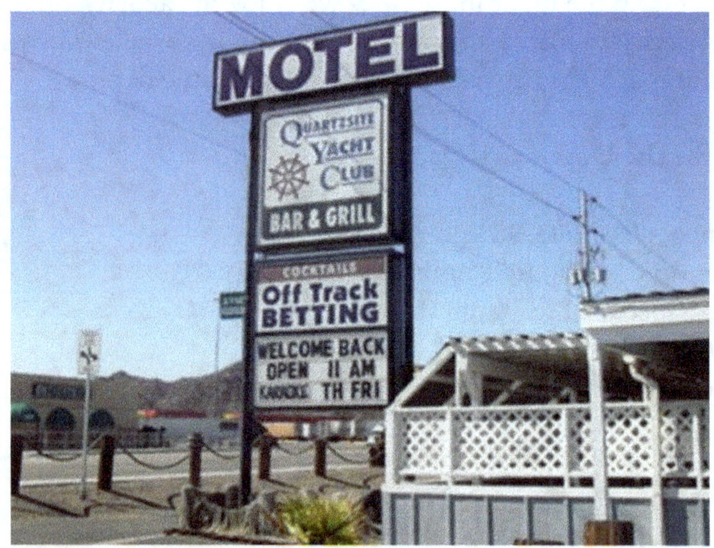

Quartzsite Yatch Club – no water, lakes, rivers, or oceans for miles.

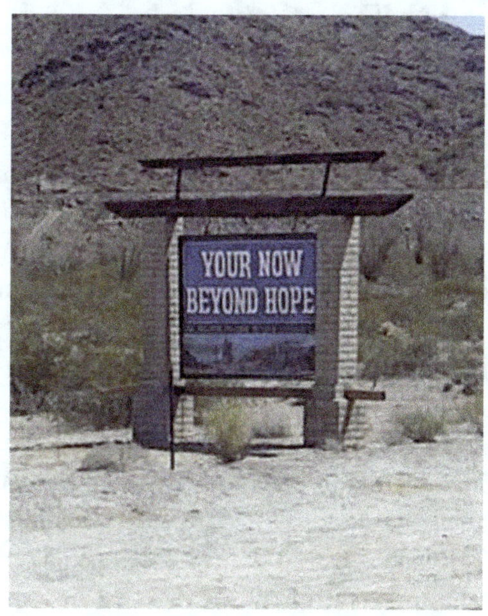

Small town of Hope, Arizona.
The sign lets you know you're now beyond hope!

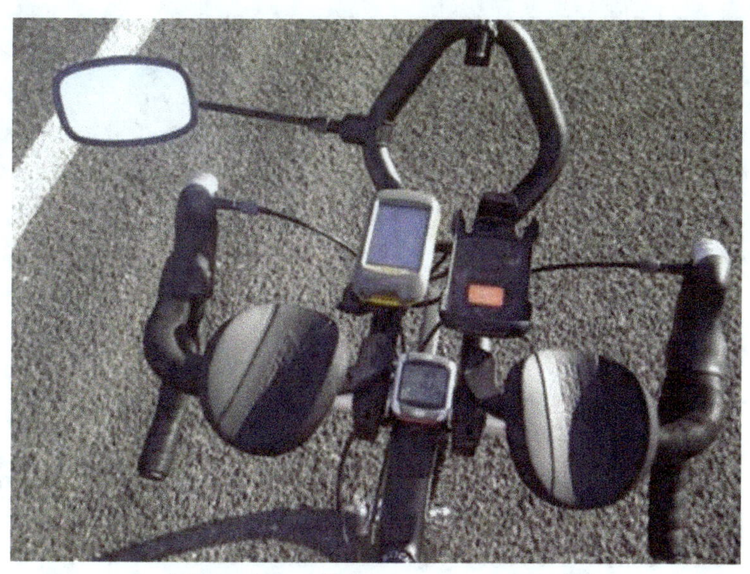

The cockpit, all the instruments needed
for a safe and informative ride.

Day 5: Monday, May 9, 2011

Salome to Wickenburg, Arizona – 62 miles/100 kilometers

Up and at it . . . the local rooster crows and this guy was right on time today. It's 5:45 a.m. and I'm thinking about a nice coffee in Wenden, the next town about 5 miles down the road. I breezed through Wenden, and this time of the morning, it's like a ghost town. So, no coffee here.

Coming into Aguilla, another small town, around 7.30 a.m., there's a bloke coming toward me pushing a loaded cart, something like a three-wheeled stroller. I moved to the other side of the road, in case he is crazy. It's people more than wild animals that are the worry out here. He says, "Any food places open down the road?"

I reply, "Yes, about 30 miles back!" We both agree this would be a good time to eat and have breakfast together at a small café.

It turns out Tony is running around the world. He's been on the road for 192 days and averages 25 miles a day! He started running across Ireland, then flew to the United States, started running from Maine, and plans to run to the bottom of South America. Then he will catch a flight to Australia and run the entire length of that, then through Asia, Middle East, and Europe on his way back to Ireland. Tony also has a few world records for ultra running. Check his website out: https://en.wikipedia.org/wiki/Tony_Mangan.

I might have freaked him out a little bit with my snake stories. Apparently he hadn't seen any so far on his run down though the United States, and he usually camped out on the side of the road at night.

I was smiling when he said he would buy me a pint of Guinness in Ireland when he finishes in six years. I wish him good luck and safe travels.

Anyhow, next stop Wickenburg, and a nice tailwind pushed me into town around noon.

I've pitched the tent and am looking forward to a BBQ under the stars for my last night of this great adventure.

Stats for the Day:

Distance – 62 miles/100 kilometers
Riding time – 4 hours 45 minutes
Average speed – 13 mph/21 kph
Elevation – 2,057 ft

The Route:

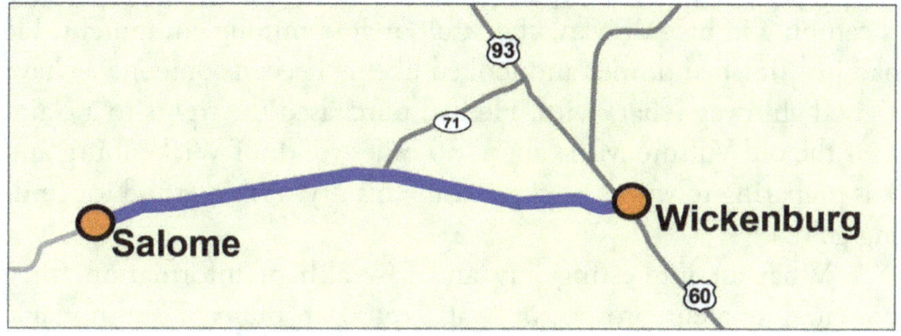

From Salome to Wickenburg, Arizona.

Picture of the Day:

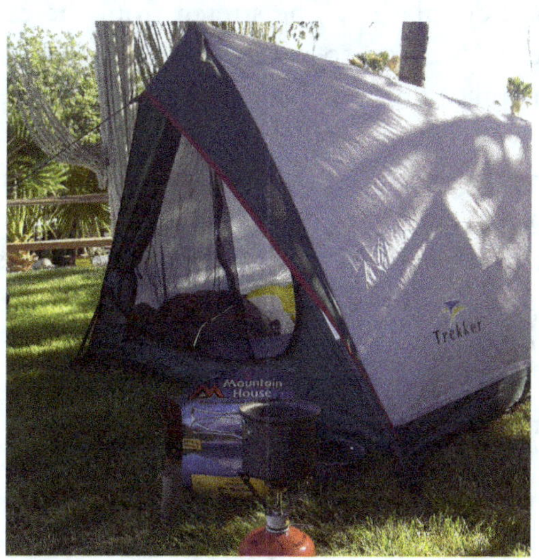

Small tent camping in Wickenburg, Arizona.

Day 6: May 10, 2011

Wickenburg to Phoenix, Arizona – 72 miles/116 kilometers

After 396 miles of cycling from San Diego, I arrive in Wickenburg, a small cowboy and prospector's town about 65 miles northwest of Phoenix. An unexpected cold snap (42°F) certainly made it a long night in the tent.

Prior to turning in for the night, I met Bill, the prospector who is camping in his minivan, chockfull of gold mining equipment. He had just finished dinner and looked like he needed someone to have a good chinwag (chat) with. He had purchased the rights to a claim near the old Vulture Mine about 30 miles south of Wickenburg and was preparing to work the claim using his dry wash method for finding gold.

What an interesting guy and a wealth of information for a potential amateur prospector – at $1,400 an ounce. Why not! He must have thought I needed a light because he came over before turning in and gave me one of his mining lights to keep as a gift.

I got going early this morning, leaving Wickenburg in the dark. This was the coldest morning so far, and it took a few good up hills to get the blood circulating. The stretch from the campsite to first coffee was about 45 miles, so halfway along, I stopped and brewed my own. What a pleasant morning, sipping a hot coffee while taking in the quietness of the surrounding bush and the tall saguaro cactus.

Not long before hitting the outskirts of Phoenix, the wind again helped speed my travels. By 11:30 a.m. I arrived at my office, then cycled to lunch at the coffee shop and made one last stop at REI to thank Tom, the mechanic, for tuning my bike prior to the ride (kind of a small victory lap). Finally, I arrived home before 2:00 p.m.

The first stage now complete, it's back to work and the start of planning the next stage of my ride in spring 2012.

Stats for the Day:

Distance – 72 miles/116 kilometers
Riding time – 6 hours 30 minutes
Average speed – 11.7 mph/18.9 kph
Elevation – 1,086 ft

The Route:

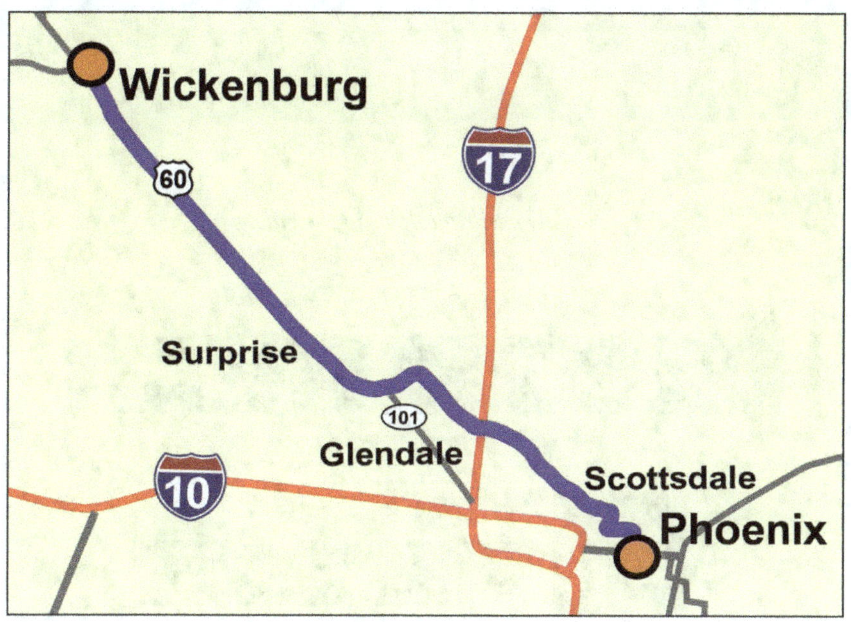

From Wickenburg to Phoenix, Arizona.

Pictures of the Day:

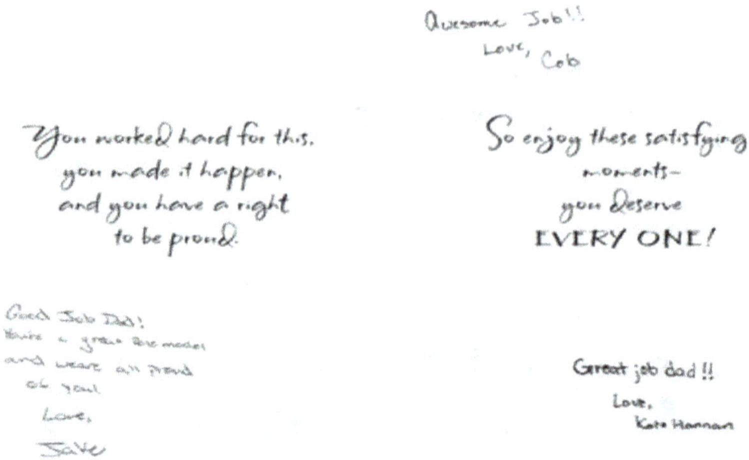

Family card to celebrate the ride.

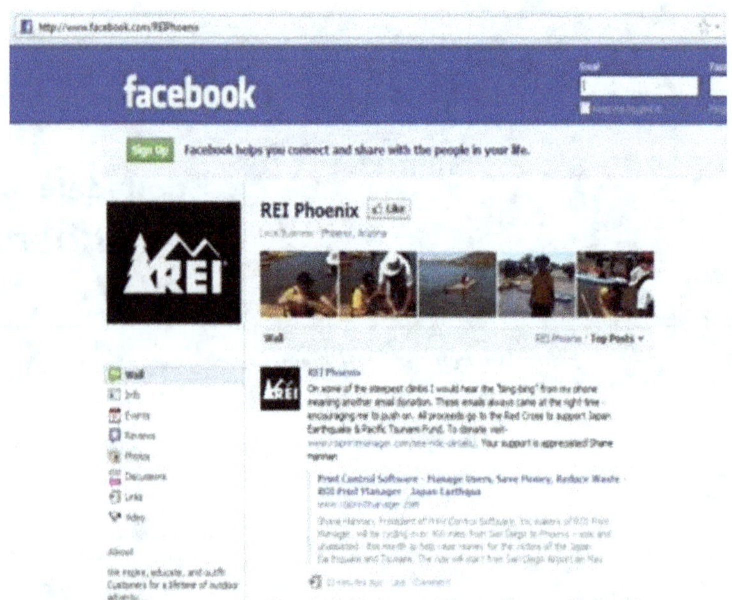

REI posted my ride on their Facebook page. They also asked me to be a guest speaker at a couple of events that reviewed the ride with other customers. I was amazed at how many people turned up to hear about my adventure.

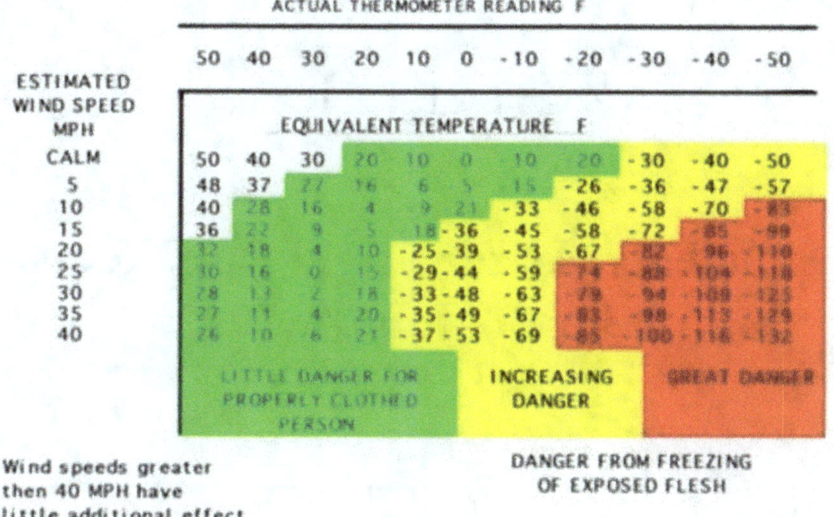

Wind Chill at 20 mph with temperature at 40°F (or 18°F or –8°C).

Footnote on the old prospector – I gave him my cell phone number to keep in contact. Well, a couple of days go by and I get a call from him. His van is stuck in the bottom of a dry creek bed. He wanted me to arrange a tow for him, which proved to be difficult and costly. So I took a drive out there next morning, found him, and towed him out of the creek. He was more than grateful and I felt happy to help him.

CHAPTER 3

Phoenix, Arizona to El Paso, Texas
May 30–June 4, 2012

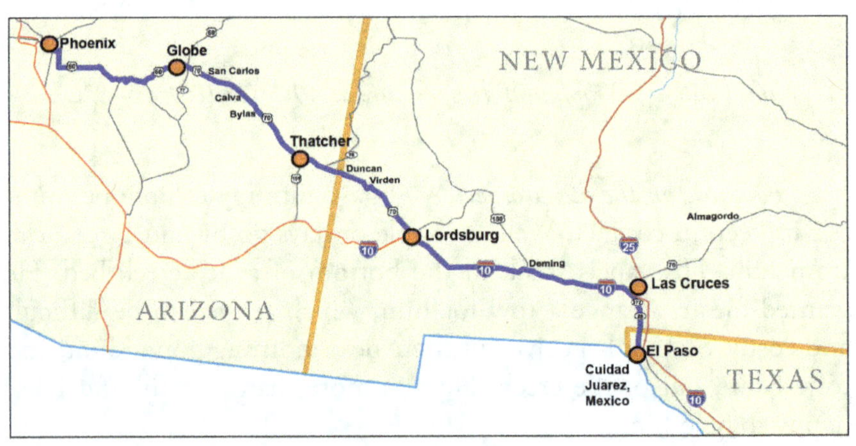

Total distance – 433 miles/700 kilometers
Number of days – 5
Average speed – 13 mph/21 kph
Total saddle time – 36 hours
Total climb – 10,059 ft/3,066 meters
Total descent – 7,346 ft/2,239 meters

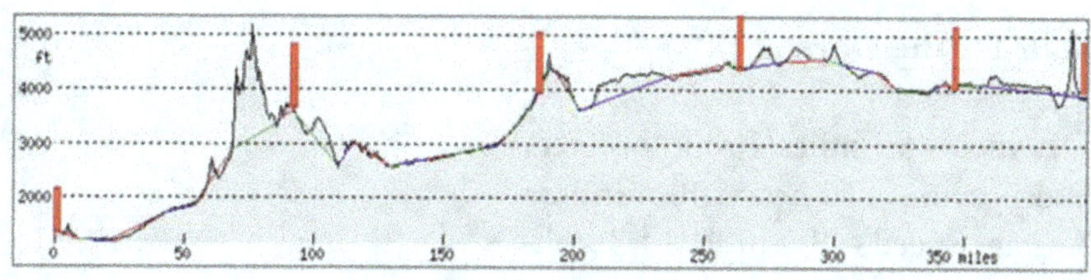

Elevation Change.

Day 1: Wednesday, May 30, 2012

Phoenix to Globe, Arizona – 98 miles/158 kilometers

How strange. I was out the front door at 4:30 a.m., in the darkness waving goodbye to Sara, thinking that in five days I would be in El Paso, Texas. The early start is to beat the traffic and heat this time of year.

At 8:00 a.m., I'm outside the metropolitan area of Phoenix and at Gold Canyon. Now the flat lands of the Phoenix valley are behind me and it's time to climb up through the Superstition Mountains. At 11:00 a.m., I arrive in Superior, which is my intended stop the first night, but it is only 11:00 a.m. and Globe is only 24 miles away – uphill. This part of the ride was the most intense I've encountered, a hot and continuous steep climb.

Passing through the Queens Creek Tunnel, about 500 yards long with no shoulder, was quite the experience. I'm at 84 miles into the ride at this point, every little pain in my body has joined as one, and I'm sweating so much, I have to stop to wipe it out of my eyes. I pass one of Sheriff Joe's chain gang crew (a.k.a. America's Toughest Sheriff) and wonder if the guard would be okay with me resting there for a bit. I keep going.

To my delight, a roadside sign states, "Next 12 Miles Download 6% Grade." But that was a lie; the downhill lasted about 2 miles. I arrived in Globe around 2:00 p.m. That was one steep hill today!

Stats for the Day:

Distance – 98 miles/158 kilometers
Riding time – 10 hours 30 minutes
Average speed – 8.9 mph/14.3 kph
Elevation – 3,510 ft

The Route:

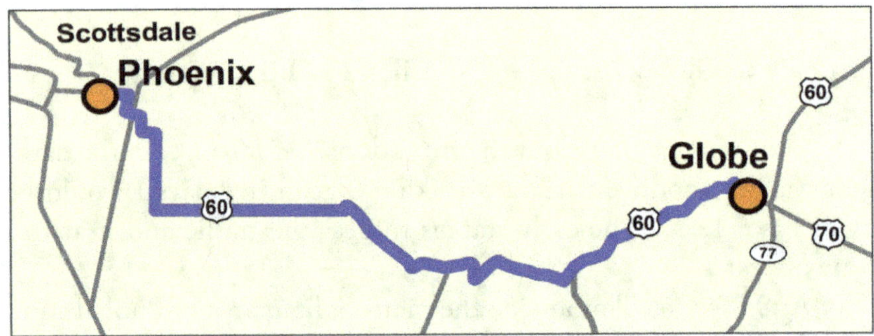

From Phoenix to Globe, Arizona.

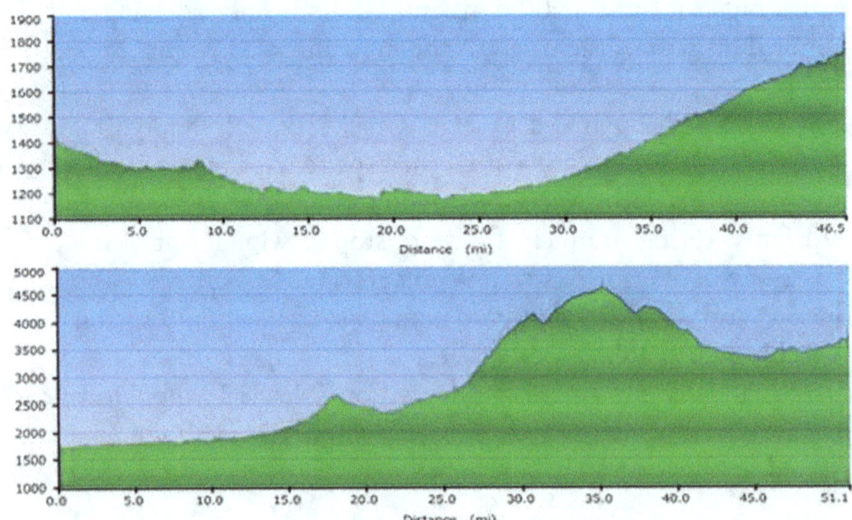

The elevation gain from Phoenix to Globe, Arizona.

Pictures of the Day:

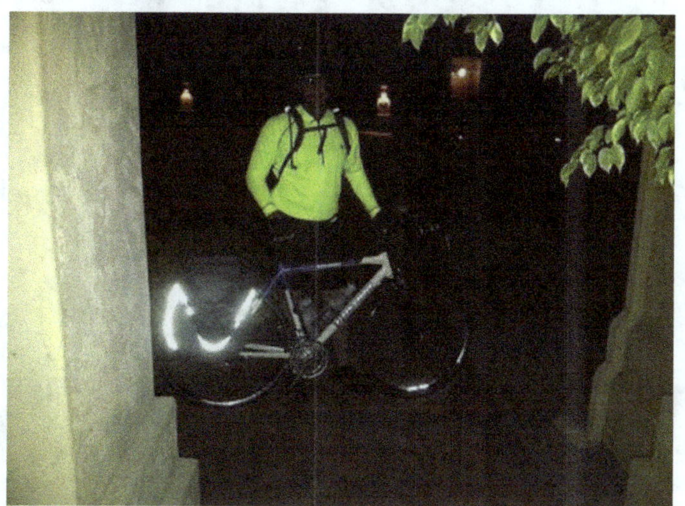

Dressed for success at 4:30 a.m.

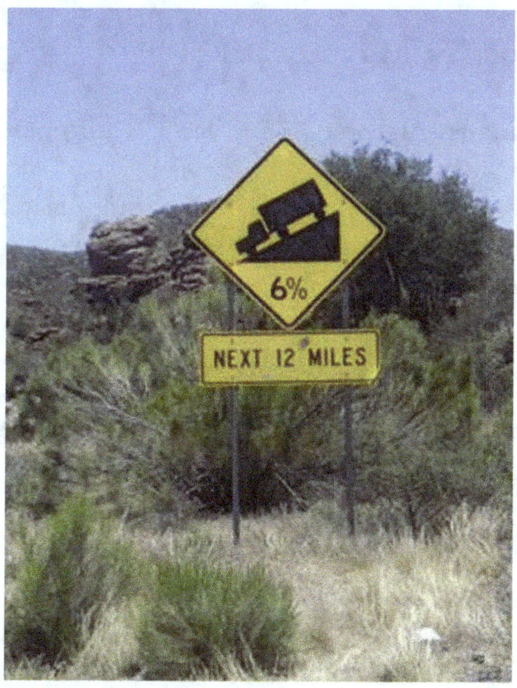

This sign is incorrect. It needs to say 2 miles, not 12 miles.

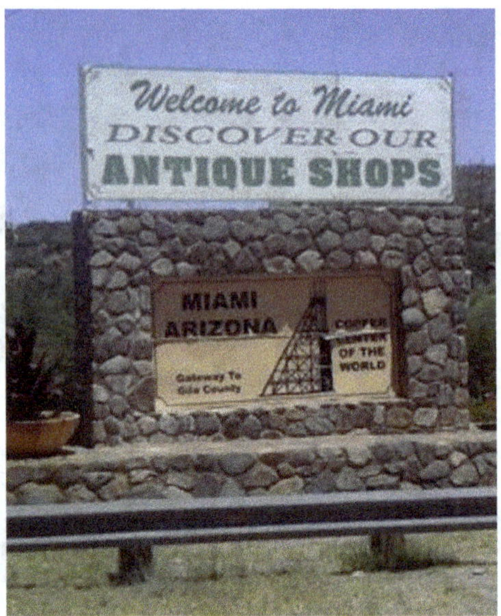

Yes, Miami, Arizona, not Miami, Florida.

Day 2: Thursday, May 31, 2012

Globe to Thatcher, Arizona – 75 miles/121 kilometers

I started around 5:30 a.m. today with some great downhill touring (top speed 42 mph) for the first 20 miles – obviously rewards from yesterday's hill climbing. Much of the morning was spent on US 70 Highway, heading southeast across the Apache Indian Reservation.

There's not much out here except miles of road and open space. Morning coffee was enjoyed on the side of the road from the camp stove with a fantastic view of the San Carlos Mountains.

These roads are now straight and long, and at times, I see mirages ahead on the road. By the time I get to where the mirage is, it turns out to be a signpost or tree. But one sighting today wasn't a mirage. Along the road in the middle of nowhere comes Rick, who is riding an elliptical scooter from South Carolina to San Diego. He's raising money for the Injured Marine Semper Fi Fund, and local fire departments are accommodating him along his route. He tells me he is seventy-one years old and it's taking him 100 days to cross the country: www.100daysforthecorps.wordpress.com.

Road conditions are good with not too much traffic and a generous shoulder. With a nice tailwind, I arrive in Thatcher, Arizona, around 11:45 a.m.

Tomorrow, Lordsburg, New Mexico!

Stats for the Day:

Distance – 75 miles/121 kilometers
Riding time – 6 hours 15 minutes
Average speed – 10.7 mph/17.2 kph
Elevation – 2,910 ft

The Route:

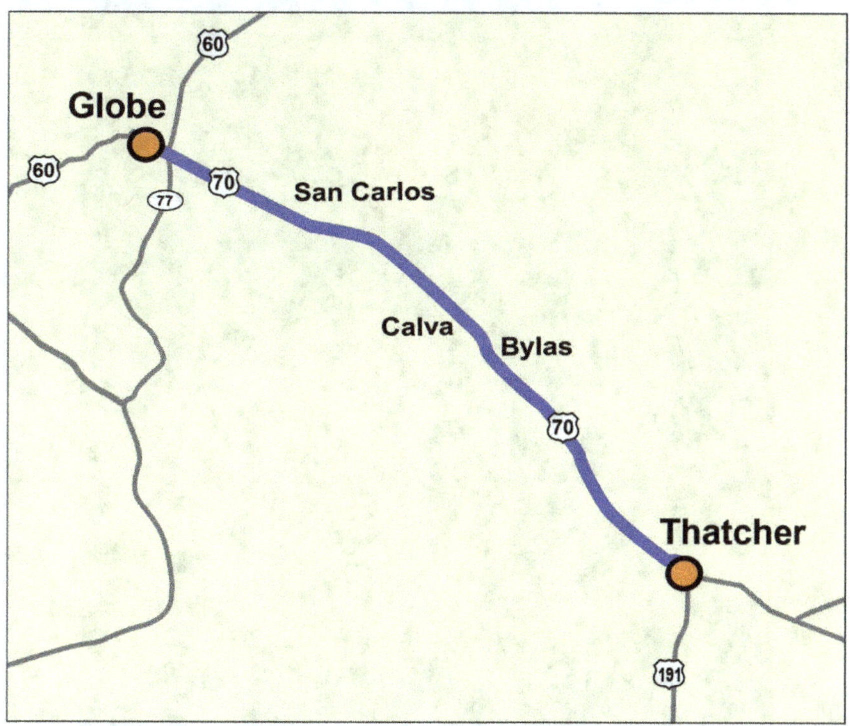

From Globe to Thatcher, Arizona.

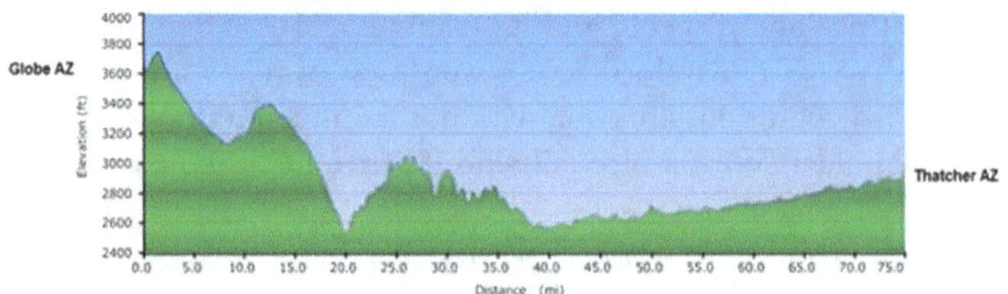

Elevation change.

Pictures of the Day:

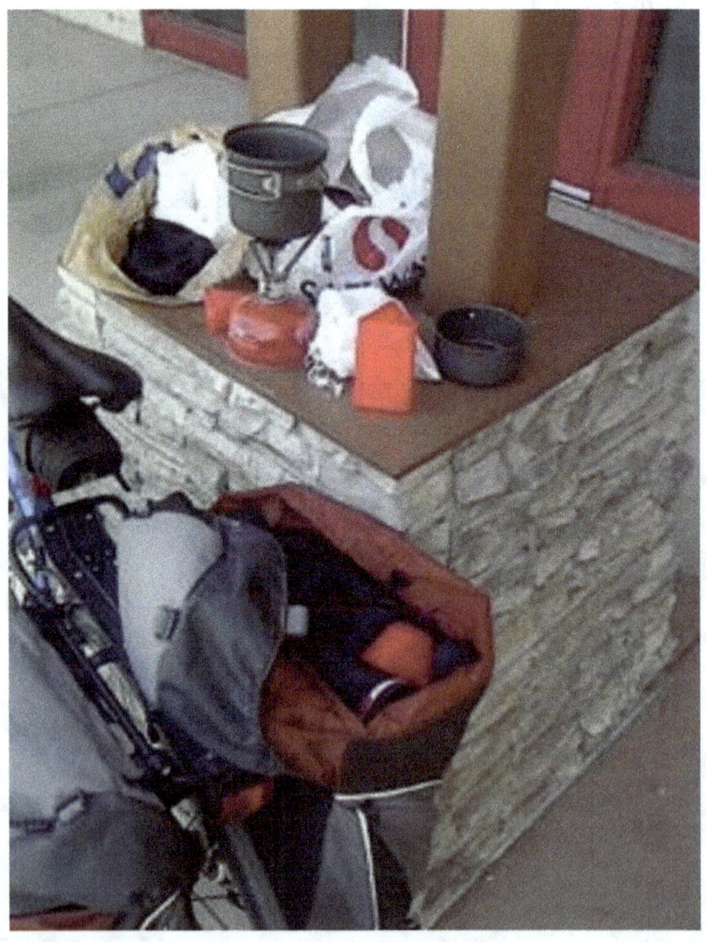

Morning coffee. Can't beat it!

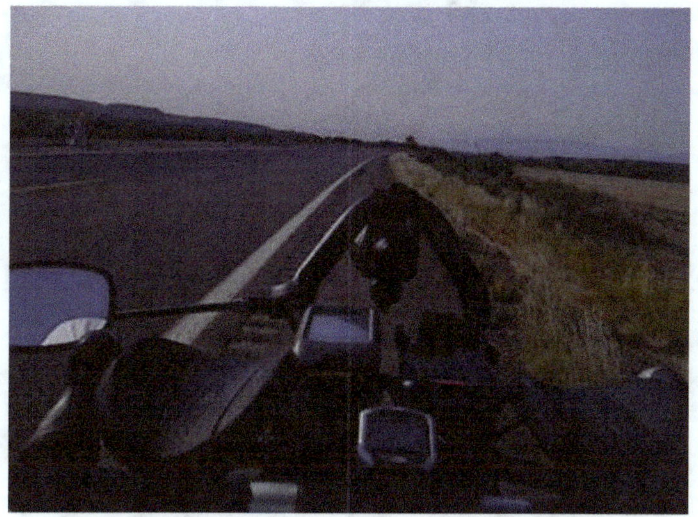

Shouldn't take photos while riding, but I did.

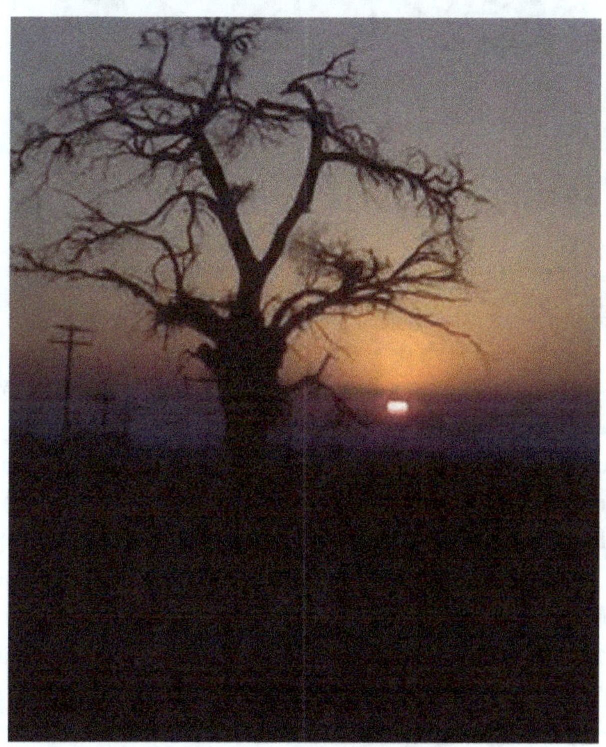

Another perfect sunrise!

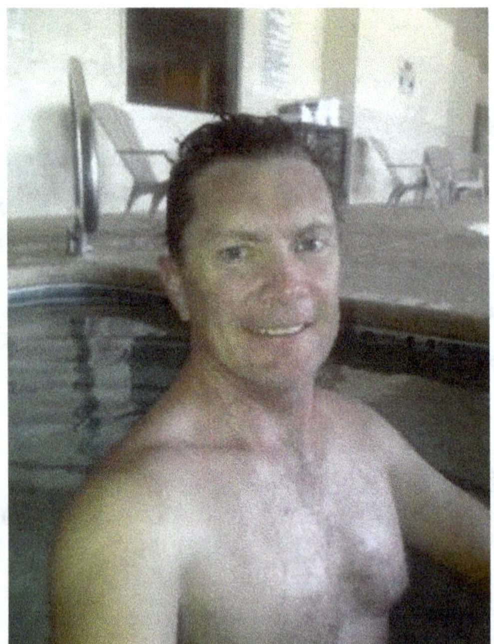

Time for a swim at the hotel.

Day 3: Friday, June 1, 2012

Thatcher, Arizona to Lordsburg, New Mexico – 80 miles/129 kilometers

I was on the road early today at 4:45 a.m. with a headwind from the southeast.

About 10 miles out of Safford, there's a zombie girl walking toward me, carrying a backpack. I remembered seeing her yesterday, walking along the main road in Thatcher. What's she doing out here in the dark, on her own, at this time of the day? I approached with caution and said, "Hi!" There is no response. I'm now within eight feet of her, and I could see her eyes weren't really focused on anything in particular, just staring off in the distance ahead. I think she mumbled something. She didn't appear distressed, so I kept on moving.

I saw my first rattlesnake this trip, crossing the road just outside Duncan, Arizona. It was a big snake taking it's time and stretched across my lane. I took to the shoulder behind it and just cycled by. Looking back, an eighteen-wheeler truck was approaching it fast. As the truck went over the snake, it must have clipped its tail. I could see the rattler lifting and twisting off the road. No need for snake pictures – I have plenty from the last trip.

It was a day of climbing and strong headwinds that slowed my progress. At the crest of each hill, there would be another hill and another. I crossed into New Mexico around 10:00 a.m. (or 11:00 a.m. NM time) and haven't encountered any aliens yet (picture attached). The roads are definitely better in Arizona/California, and again, it's quite open out here. There's nothing (nothing!) for miles – just long stretches of road that disappear into the horizon and open desert on either side that runs up to the base of the mountains. I can't imagine how long it would have taken people to cross this terrain on horses with no roadways. One historical marker tells the story of two settlers who were killed by Indians over two hundred years ago at this spot. Creepy, better keep riding just in case.

I arrived in Lordsburg at 11:45 a.m. (AZ time) and headed straight to McDonald's for a bacon ranch salad with crispy chicken, followed by a quarter pounder with chips.

I was planning on heading south from Lordsburg to Columbus, New Mexico, and follow the US-Mexico border into El Paso, Texas, but the locals advised me to stick with Interstate 10 via Deming to Las Cruces. There are plenty of potential problems with this route: illegal border activities, long stretches without service or shade, and a lone bicyclist – not a good combination! Interstate 10 has service stops about every 20 miles. So tomorrow it's Deming, New Mexico.

Stats for the Day:

Distance – 80 miles/129 kilometers
Riding time – 6 hours 30 minutes
Average speed – 12.3 mph/19.8 kph
Elevation – 4,249 ft

The Route:

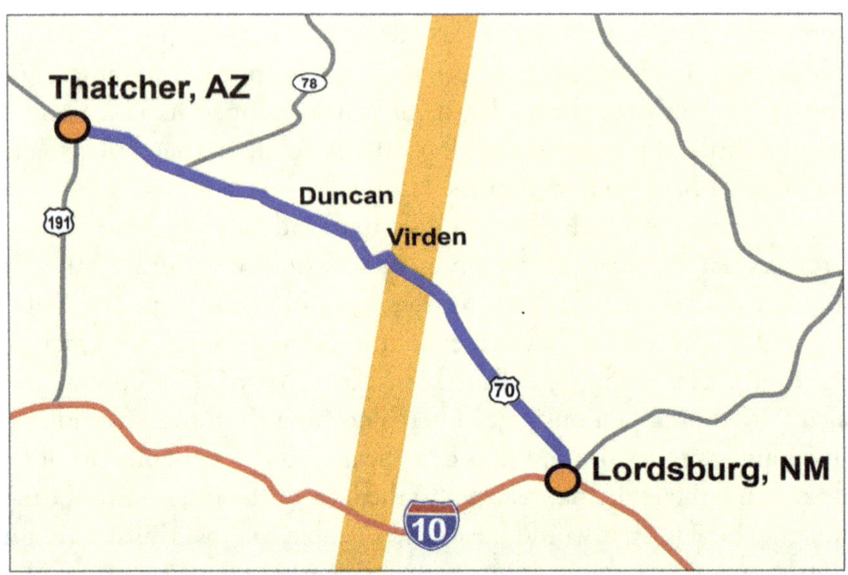

From Thatcher, Arizona, to Lordsburg, New Mexico.

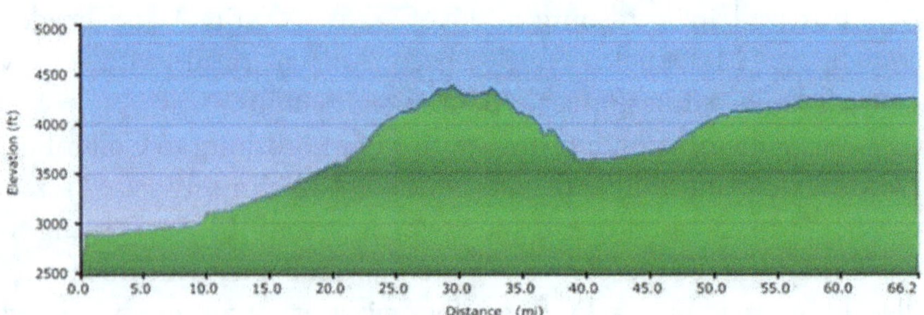

Elevation change.

Picture of the Day:

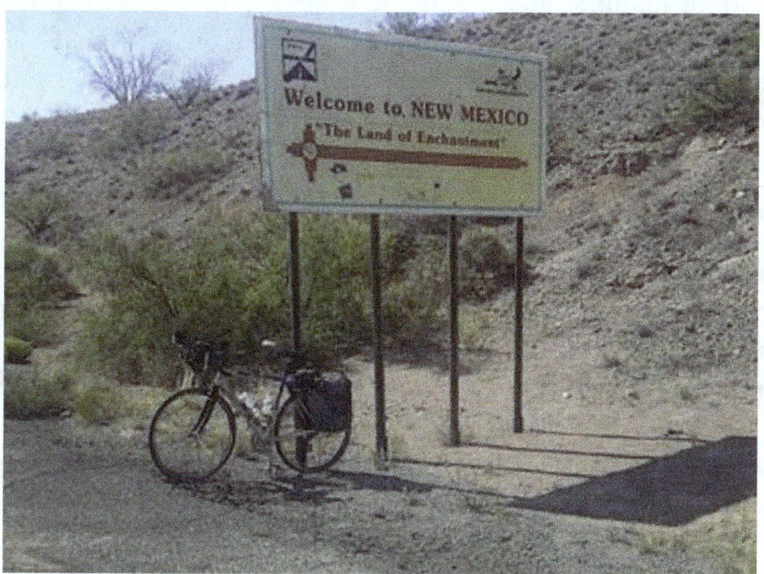

The border between Arizona and New Mexico.

Day 4: Saturday, June 2, 2012

Lordsburg to Las Cruces, New Mexico – 124 miles/200 kilometers

Pump it up! That's all I heard in my head today! My legs pumped hard (124 miles from Lordsburg, NM, to Las Cruces, NM) *and* I spent a lot of time pumping up flat tires – *five* rear wheel changes to be exact!

I left Lordsburg at daylight, around 5:15 a.m., and the first 63 miles were on Interstate 10 to Deming, NM, where I was planning on staying the night. It was Saturday morning, and although traffic was light, there were still plenty of trucks. Within the first fifteen minutes this morning, I had a flat tire on the back wheel. I could feel it go – a sharp stone on the wrong angle. There's no way around it. I had to take the luggage off, lay the bike flat in the dirt, and fix it. The side of the freeway was like a pool table and required plenty of concentration to maneuver around the obstacles on the shoulder lane.

No more than ten minutes later, another flat on the rear! You have to be kidding. This is going to be a great day! On closer inspection, the tire has a small piece of wire sticking out. My mate Ralph, back in Phoenix, warned me this would be a problem. Interstate 10 in this area is known to cause many cyclists to become expert tire repairers. The punctures are caused by the debris from truck tires that contain wire.

The journey continues – and another flat. Same deal, a small piece of wire again. Fix it and move on. I knew it would be bad, but there's no alternative. On the fifth flat, I replaced the tire with a spare I was carrying and made it into Butterfield Station. I'm completely demoralized by now, thinking about the road ahead and more flat tires.

I'm covered in dust and have grease on my hands from the chain; it's just about everywhere on me. I look like I've been riding a mountain bike through the desert and came off a few times.

A sign at the gas station catches my eye: "Las Cruces 80 Miles." Now I'm inspired. Forty miles done, eighty miles to go. I think I can make that! I get to Deming, which is 20 more miles, without a problem. While there, I patch my tubes and get cleaned up. I repair four tubes with patches, and I'm really hoping the next 60 miles are free of punctures.

It's time for breakfast at the gas station in Deming, and a chat with the locals about alternatives to Interstate 10. "There's nothing between here and Las Cruces except the I-10," Pops says from behind the cash register. While having breakfast, I find a tourist map and an alternative route to the Interstate which is Highway 549. This takes me away from the interstate for about 25 miles, then meets up again, and turns out to be a perfect back road – no problem and no trucks. The road is long and flat, disappearing into a mirage up ahead. Is that a biker I see ahead coming my way? Turns out to be another signpost.

The Interstate 10 is about 3 miles to my left. The trucks move in silence and look like caterpillars following each other. Eventually I meet back up with Interstate 10 at Akela Flats (funny name "flats"). I buy an ice cream and take a tour of the gas station store. The girl behind the counter informs me that Highway 549 will take me another 15 miles along before having to get on the Interstate 10 again. Nice!

At 100 miles done, I've only got 24 miles to go on the interstate. I arrive in Las Cruces at 3:15 p.m. That's ten hours and now I'm really ready for a cold one, or three! Tonight's dinner is at Luna Rossa Winery and Pizza. I highly recommend it if you are passing through here sometime.

Final day tomorrow – 50 miles to El Paso, Texas.

Stats for the Day:

Distance – 124 miles/200 kilometers
Riding time – 10 hours
Average speed – 12 mph/19.3 kph
Elevation – 3,900 ft

The Route:

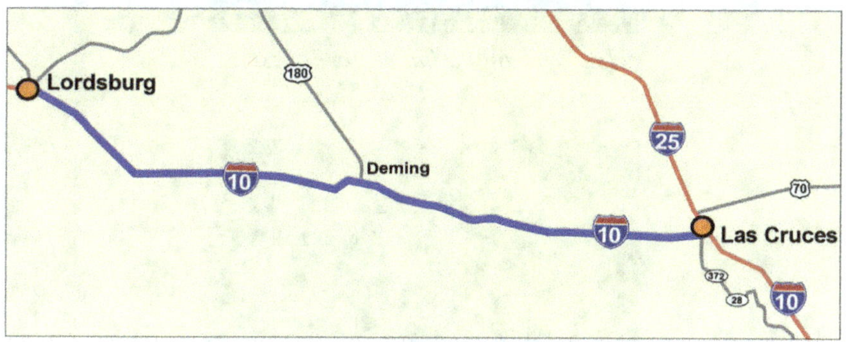

From Lordsburg to Las Cruces, New Mexico.

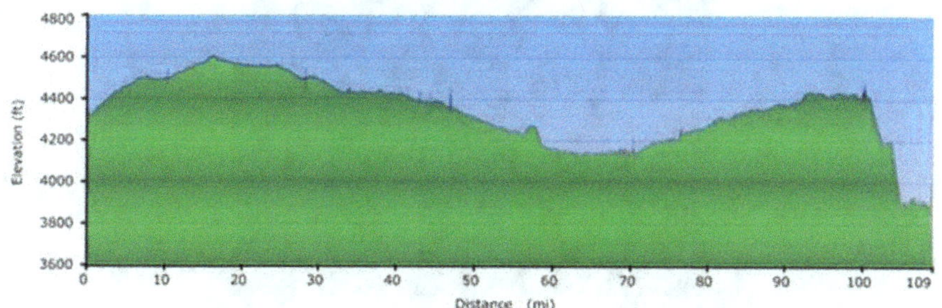

Elevation change.

Pictures of the Day:

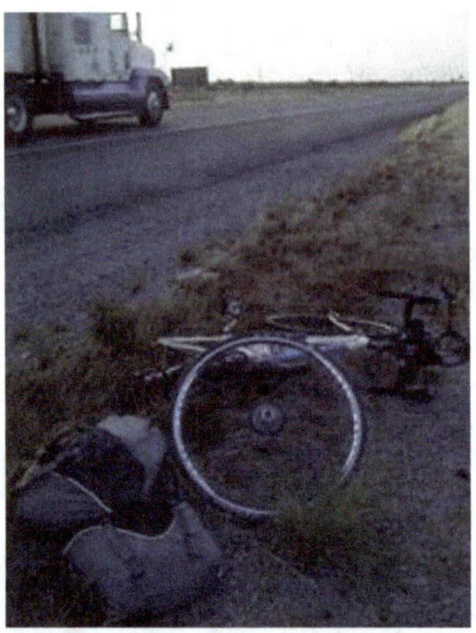

How to change a flat on the interstate.

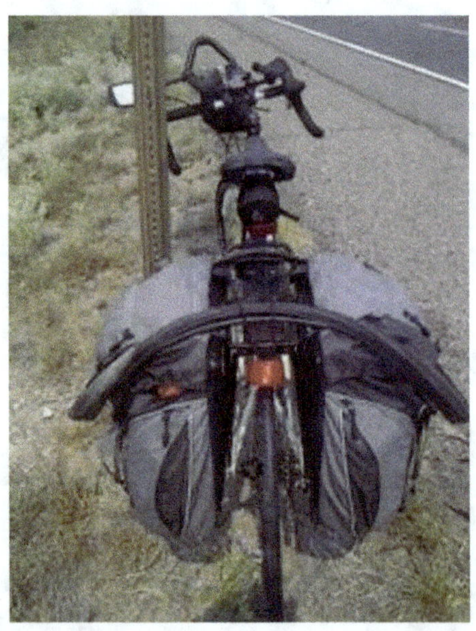

Didn't want to litter so carried the old tire.

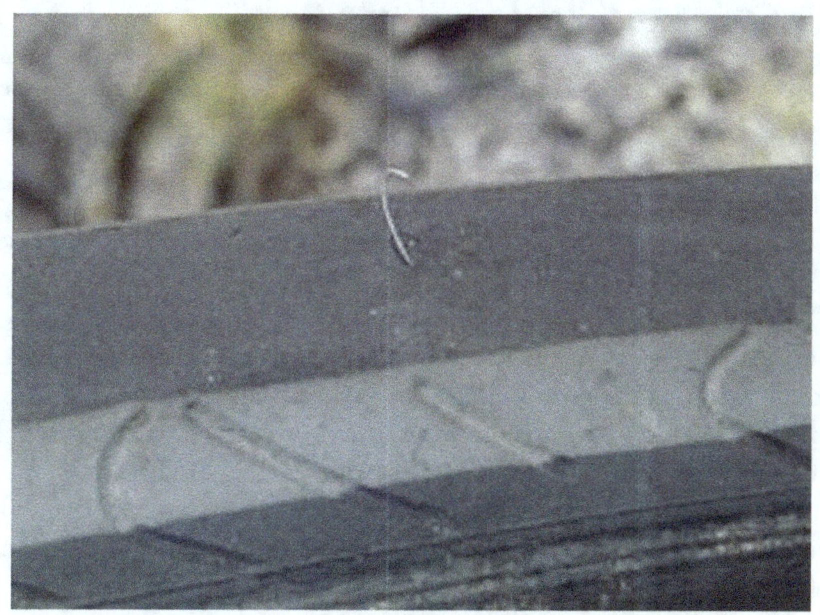

I know, but this a different flat in a different location.

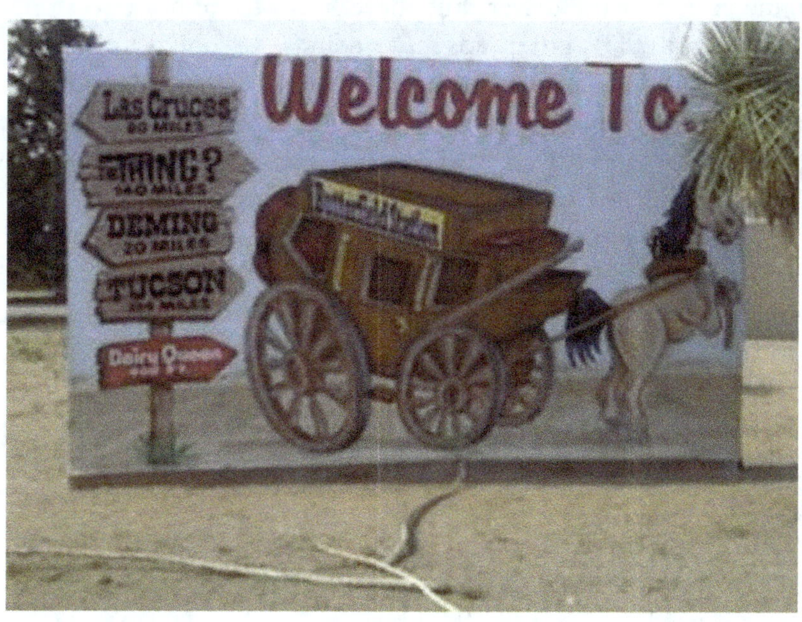

A sign of inspiration – only 80 miles to go after a tough morning.

Day 5: June 3, 2012

Las Cruces, New Mexico to El Paso, Texas – 53 miles/85 kilometers

Well rested from yesterday's marathon ride, it was an easy Sunday morning cycle from Las Cruces to El Paso, a total of 53 miles. The route follows the Rio Grande (Big River) for most of the ride. This river starts in southern Colorado and cuts through the center of New Mexico, then follows the US-Mexico border along the bottom of Texas. The river provides water for all the farming in this area. Pecan tree farms and other crops lined either side of the road before I crossed into Texas, around 10:30 a.m. From there, it was light traffic through downtown El Paso, and I finished the ride around 11:45 a.m.

There is always something that happens when you are on a bicycle adventure, and today was no different. In El Paso, a bunch of cars stopped on the road with people running everywhere. As I approached, the hood was up on one of the cars with a person under it. Strange. It turns out that a kitten had crawled up into the car's engine area, and the driver must have heard some noise so stopped the car, luckily. The kitten was rescued and everyone is fine.

I checked into the hotel and the luggage that I sent ahead is waiting for me. I boxed up my carry-on roller bag with my business suits, and had it FedEx'd to the final hotel. Tomorrow I will have meetings with the local dealers who sell my software.

Now, back in civilization I need a car, so I ride to the airport a few miles from the hotel and pick up a rental, then go to the local bike shop for an empty bike box. Back at the hotel, I pack up my bike and riding gear, ready for the flight back to Phoenix tomorrow evening.

Next leg – El Paso, Texas, to San Antonio Texas!

Stats for the Day:
Distance – 53 miles / 85 kilometers
Riding Time – 4.30 hours
Average Speed – 12 mph / 19.3 kph
Elevation – 3,740 ft

The Route:

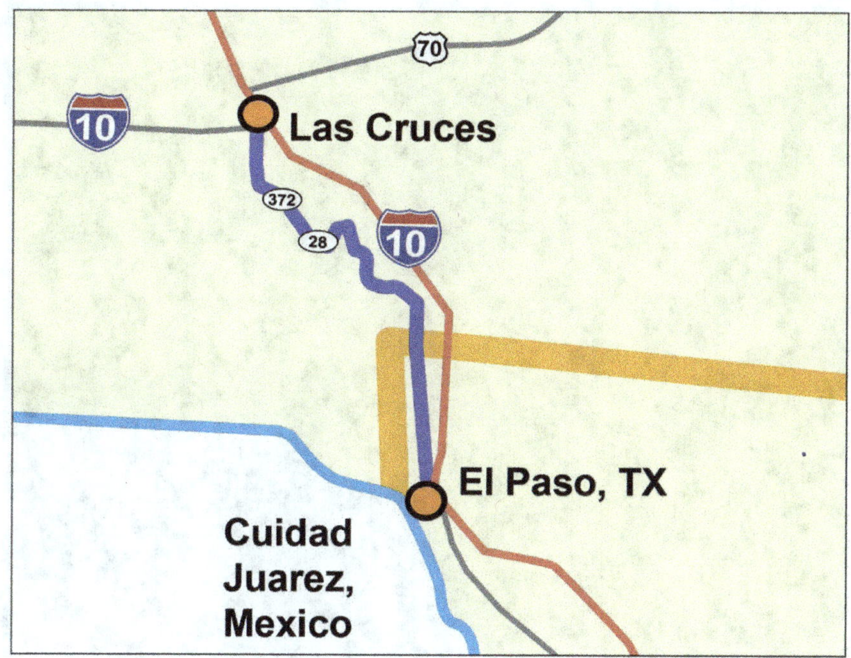

From Las Cruces, New Mexico, to El Paso, Texas

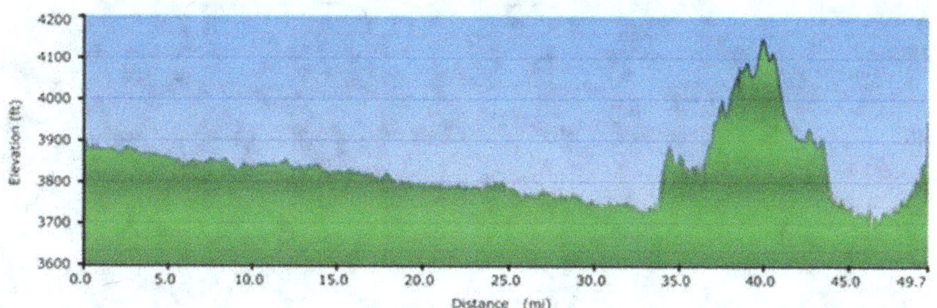

Elevation change.

Pictures of the Day:

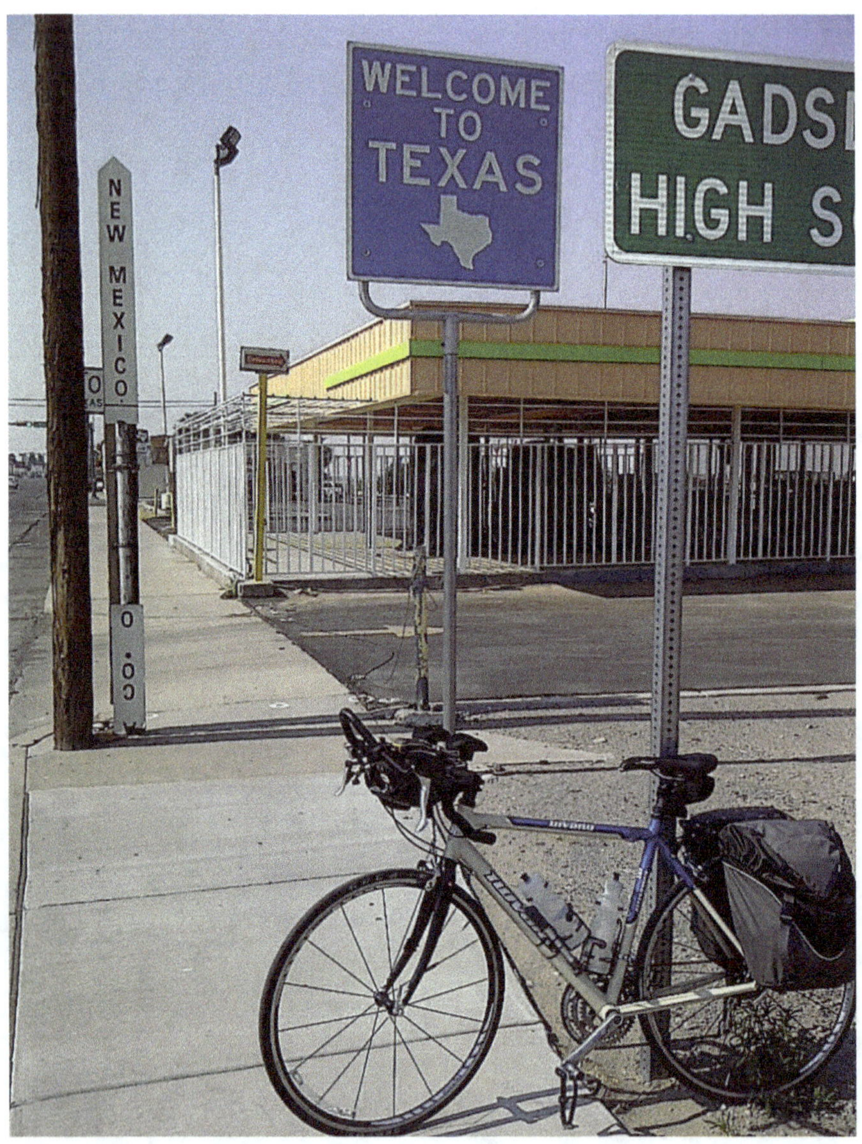

On the boarder of New Mexico and Texas.

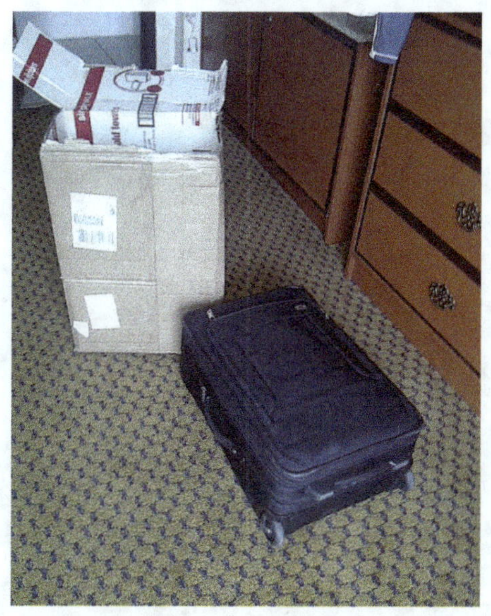

My roller bag with business attire FedEx'ed from Phoenix.

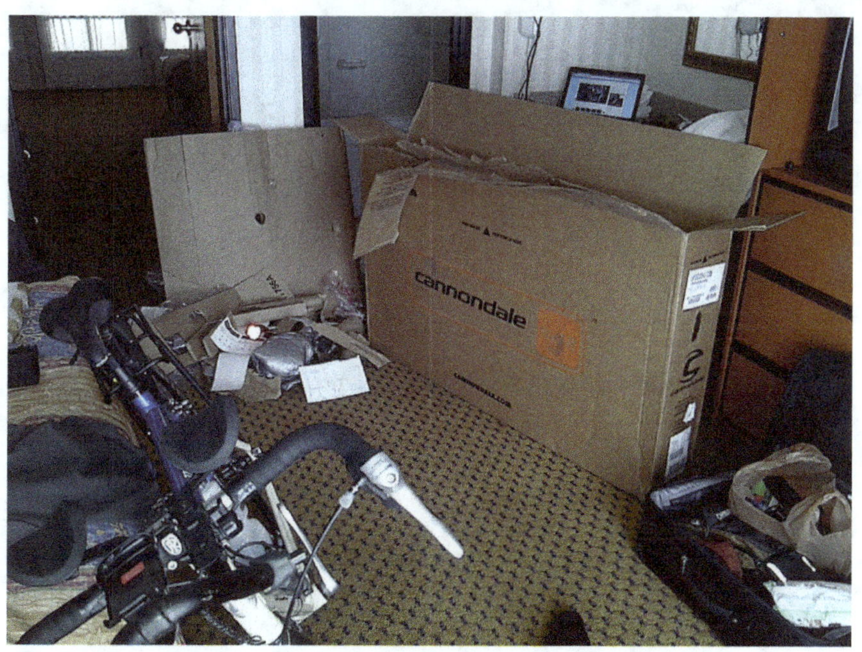

Packing my bike for the flight back to Phoenix.

CHAPTER 4

El Paso, Texas to San Antonio, Texas
May 2–May 8, 2013

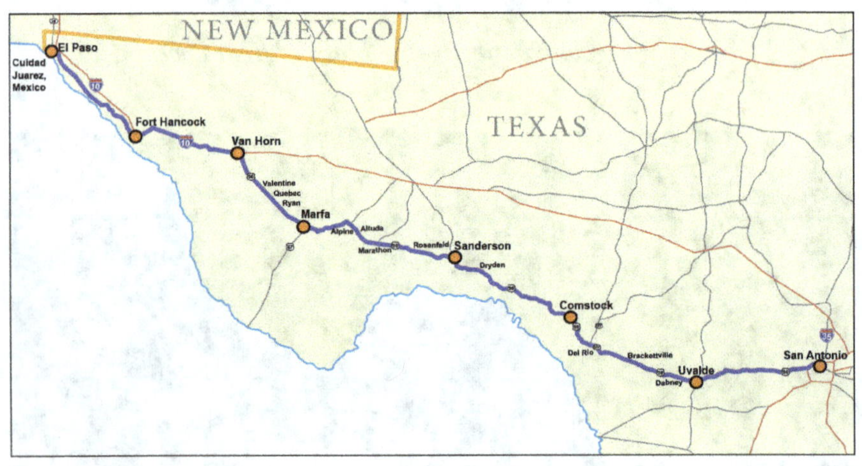

Total distance – 620 miles/1,000 kilometers
Number of days – 7
Average speed – 12.4 mph/20 kph
Total saddle time – 50 hours

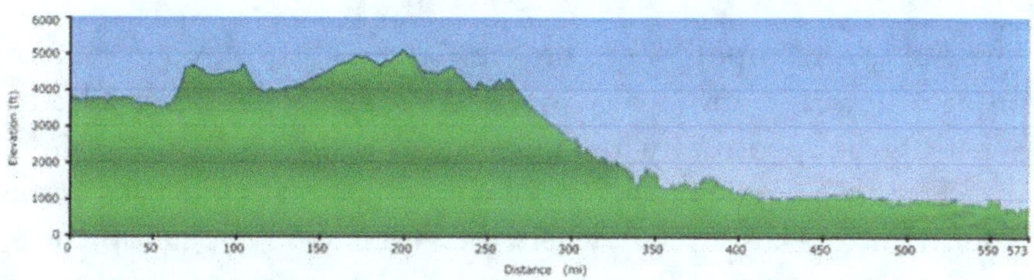

Day 1: Thursday, May 2, 2013

El Paso to Fort Hancock – 54 miles/87 kilometers

Early start – 6:20 a.m. flight from Phoenix Sky Harbor airport. At the Southwest Airlines check in, the agent gets me again for a $75 oversize luggage fee for my bike. I just accept the fee because I know that when I call the airline's customer service center they will credit this fee back. They have me on file and see my progress as I book flights with the same airline for the ride.

Arrival into El Paso was on time at 8.30 a.m. Mountain Standard Time, followed by a quick change into my bike clothes. The Southwest Airline guys carry my boxed bike to me for assembly in the baggage claim area. They ask where I'm going. "San Antonio," I tell them.

One of them responds with, "That's a long way!"

I tell them, "I thought it was just a day's cycle, maybe 70 miles."

"No," he responds, "it's almost 700 miles!" Next thing, I have a curious crowd asking all types of questions ("You rode from *Australia*?").

The airport was fairly empty that time of day. After about thirty minutes I have everything packed, bike back together and ready to go. I ride in the baggage claim area over to the Southwest customer services counter and thank them for getting rid of the bike box. They insist on a picture with me standing behind their counter and invite me to join them in September for a seventy-mile ride to help the USO from Fort Bliss.

Wow! That cold front from Canada really took the temperatures down. It was 46°F and windy heading out of the airport. At the entrance to the airport was a bronze statue of a giant conquistador riding a horse. It was as big, well almost, as the Statue of Liberty. What a great opportunity for a photo.

First thing was a quick breakfast at McDonald's, then across the road to Crazy Cats Cyclery where they were good enough to check my tire pressure and inflate as needed. The storeowner said she sees twenty people a day this time of year, coming by the store, bicycling their way across the US.

After negotiating my way through downtown heading east, I was pretty much following the Mexican border all day. The town on the other side of the border is Ciudad Juarez, known for drug cartels and drug trafficking.

The wind got stronger in the afternoon and at one point blew me off the road surface into the gravel shoulder. I was lucky not to come off the bike. Imagine riding at eight miles per hour with a side wind / headwind gusting to forty miles per hour and plenty of dust. That was my day. I finished around 3:30 p.m. at the Fort Hancock Motel. Right across the road from the hotel is Angie's World Famous Chicken Fried Steak Restaurant, and it lived up to their claim!

After dinner, I was lucky enough to discuss tomorrow's route with the local sheriff, and his suggestions were very helpful. He made a hand drawn map on a bar coaster. Instead of taking the shoulder of Interstate 10, his recommendation was to take TX 20 to Farm to Market Number 192 Road for about 12 miles, then turn left onto Farm to Market Road Number 34. This would bring me out at mile marker 92 on Interstate 10. This is a great way to avoid the trucks on the highway and only ride about two miles on the interstate until I reach the access road which runs all the way to Allamoore. Luckily, there was a napkin close by that he used to write out the directions.

Stats for the Day:

Distance – 54 miles/87 kilometers
Riding time – 4 hours 15 minutes
Average speed – 12.7 mph/20.4 kph
Elevation – 3,515 ft

The Route:

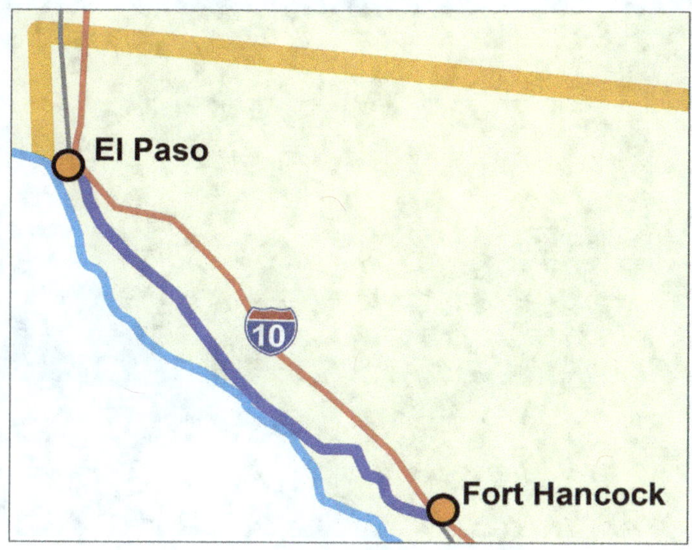

From El Paso to Fort Hancock, Texas.

Pictures of the Day:

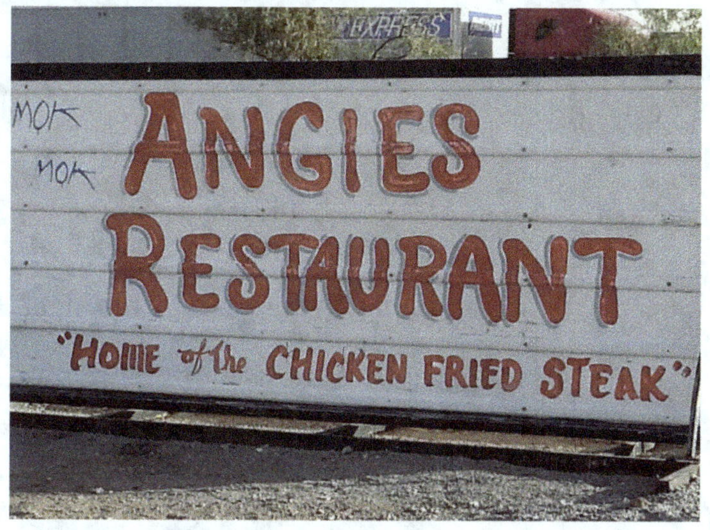

Angie's Restaurant – exit 148 off the Interstate 10.
Just north of the Mexico Boarder.

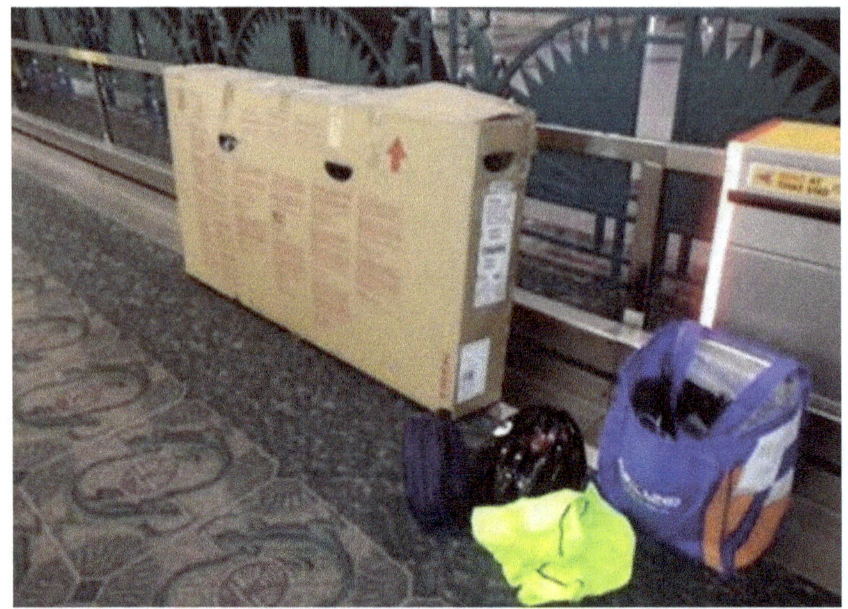

Baggage claim at El Paso Airport.

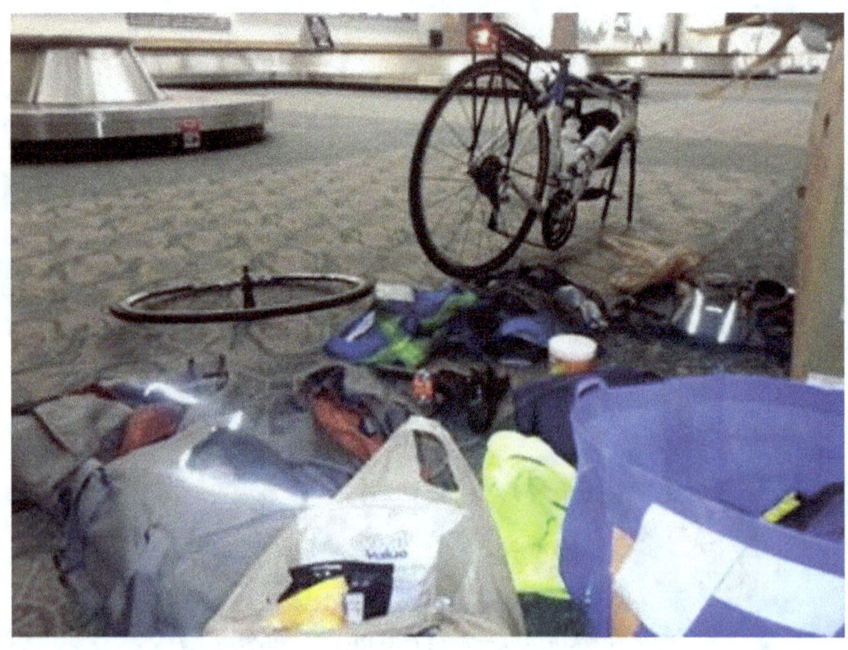

A little messy while getting things organized.

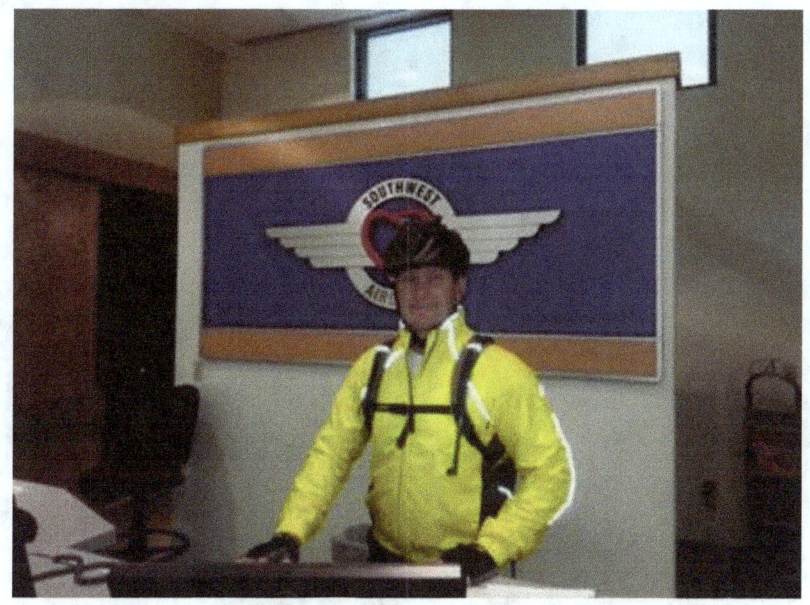

Southwest Airlines agent wanted a pic from her desk.

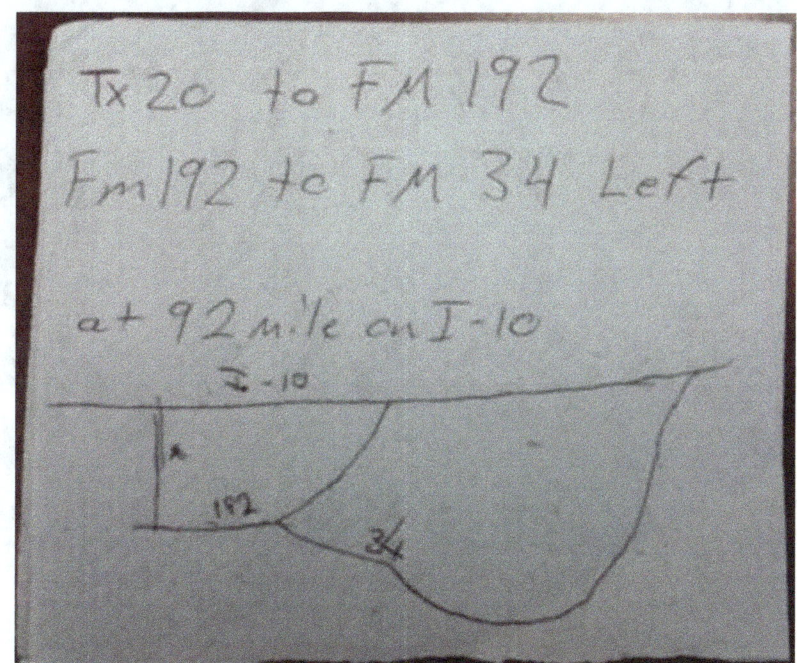

Sheriff's helpful directions on a napkin.

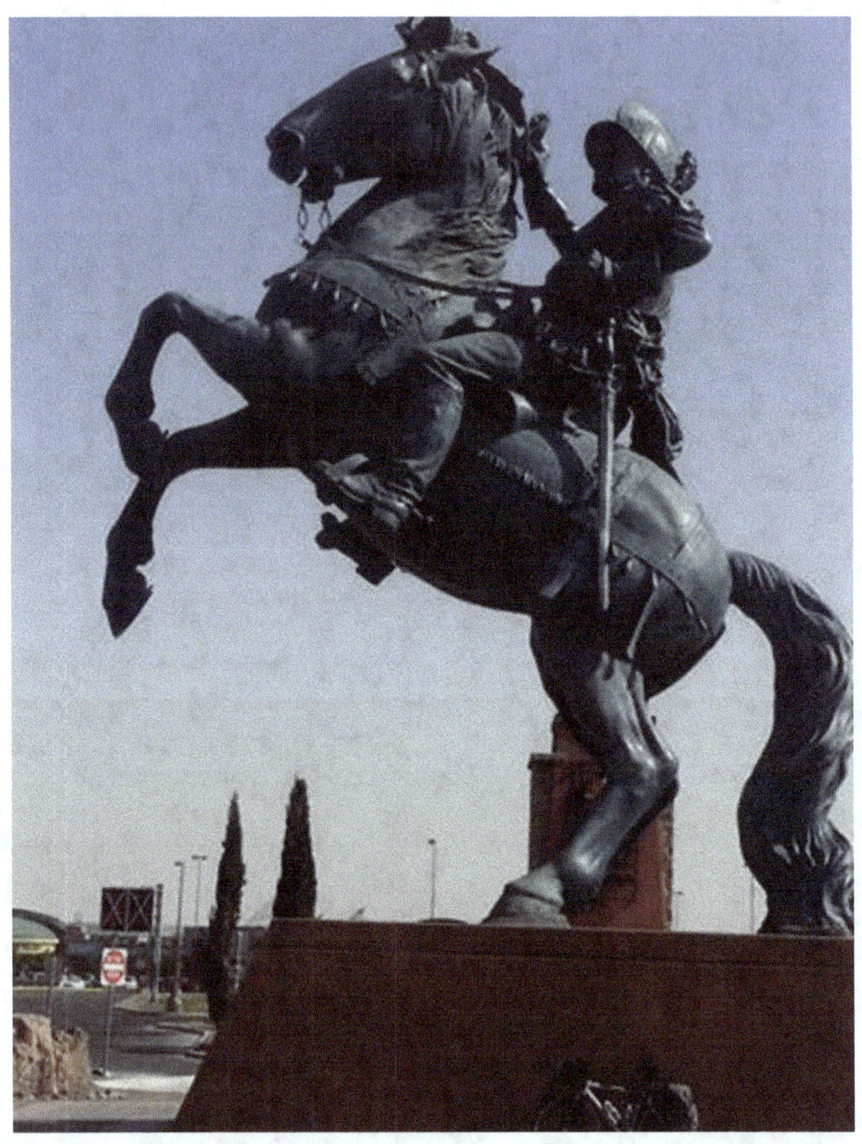

Outside El Paso Airport – giant conquistador or small bike.

Day 2: Friday, May 3, 2013

Fort Hancock to Van Horn – 77 miles/124 kilometers

I had a great breakfast at Angie's at 6:00 a.m.: bacon, eggs, toast, and coffee with the locals. It was cold out this morning (36°F, or 2°C), so I wore both sets of bike clothes until the temperature reached 55°F (13°C). I was on the road today at 6:40 a.m., taking the back way around Interstate 10 for about 25 miles, all along farmland that bordered Mexico. This was a great test for my new Continental Gatorskin tires because the road was all loose gravel. I made my way back to the interstate and started on the climb, which was basically the rest of the day along with the headwind, but not as bad as yesterday.

After a few miles, I joined a frontage road along Interstate 10 that took me all the way to Allamoore. It was time to make a decision – take Interstate 10 or go the back road and follow Google Maps? I take the back road that is dirt for the first 1,000 feet, then follow the train line for about half a mile, only to be stopped at a gate that reads "No Trespassing." So back to the Interstate 10.

I'm now about ten miles from Van Horn and still pushing uphill. Then about six miles along, I can start to see the trucks ahead finally disappear on the crest of the next hill. It was downhill for the last 4 miles into Van Horne.

I finished this day at 2:30 p.m. I'm now in the Central Time Zone. These roads are long and straight in West Texas. It's no bicycle ride through the wine country, that's for sure!

Some people ask me if my bum gets sore sitting on the saddle for such a long time each day.

And yes, it does, but only when I'm not enjoying the ride, which is when there's a headwind or a long hill climb or both at the same time. There is never any pain when going down a hill or having the wind at my back or both at the same time.

Another question from Pierre, who lives in Paris, "Isn't it too difficult along these long roads?" Answer? Same as above.

Richard (the Aussie I met on Day 3 in California) you were right about the Cattle Company Steak House in Van Horne. It *is* great. I just got back from dinner and the rib eye steak was awesome!

Stats for the Day:

Distance – 77 miles/124 kilometers
Riding time – 6 hours 25 minutes
Average speed – 11.9 mph/19.2 kph
Elevation – 4,139 ft.

The Route:

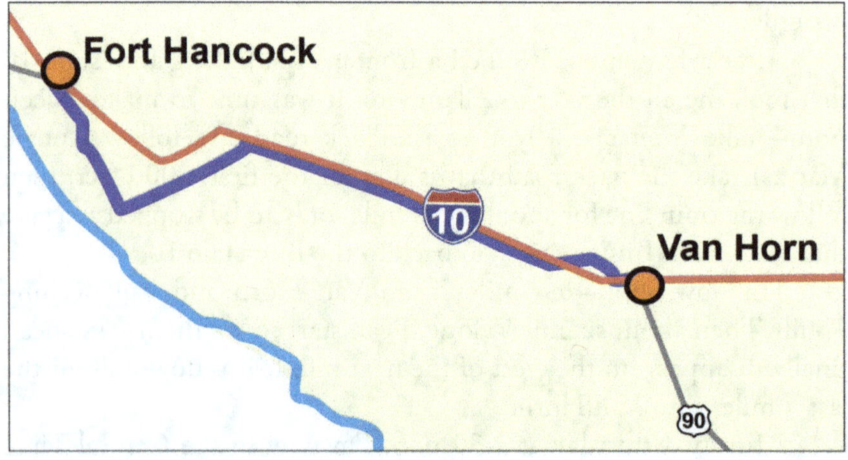

From Fort Hancock to Van Horn, Texas.

Pictures of the Day:

Makes it all worth it!

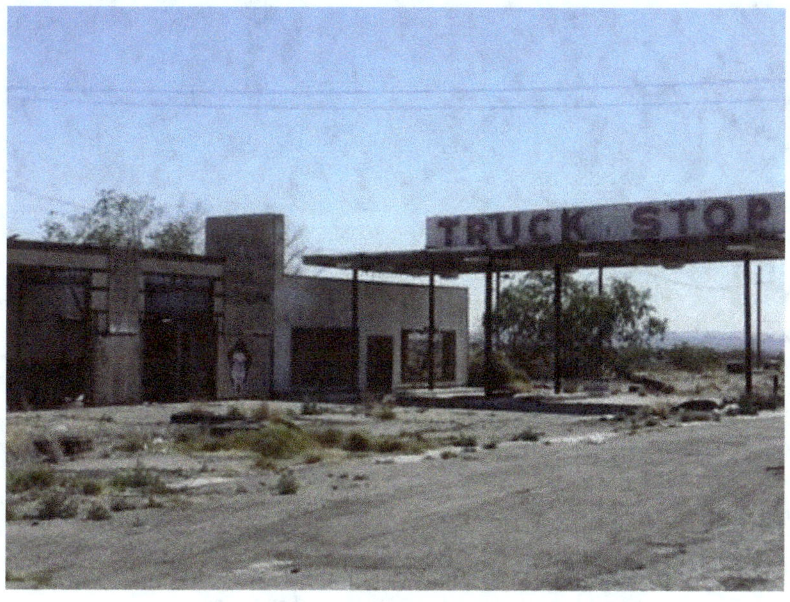

Sierra Blanca, Texas – a ghost town.

71

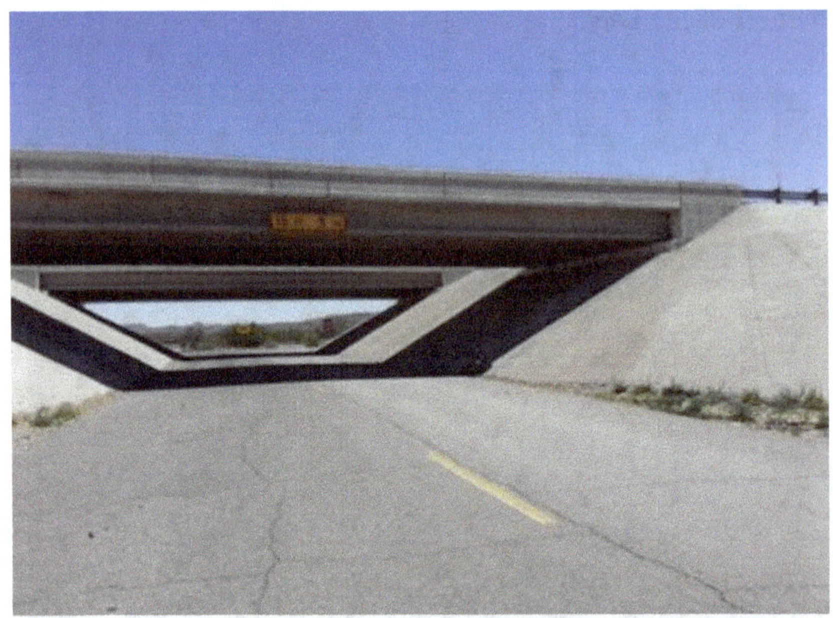

Lunch under the Interstate 10.

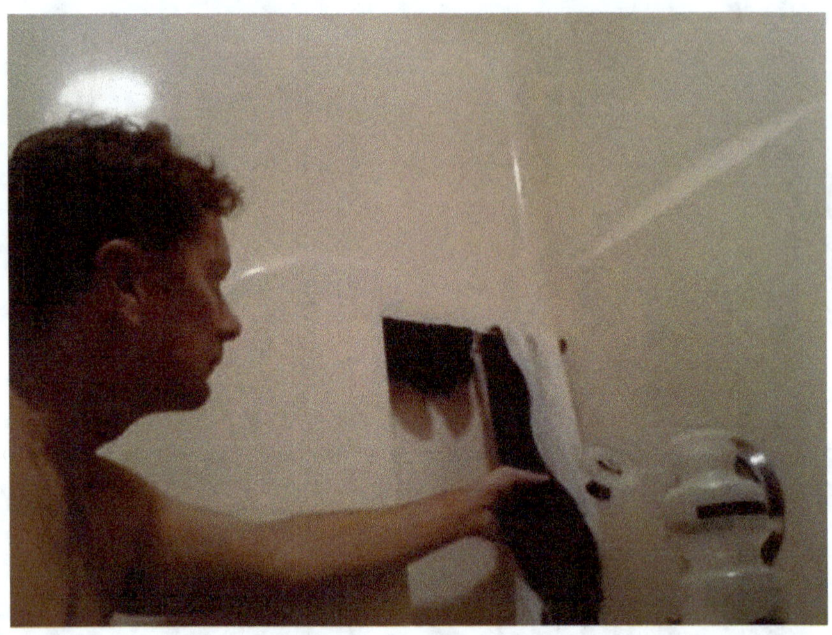

The nightly routine — bath and wash clothes.

Day 3: Saturday, May 4, 2013

Van Horn to Marfa – 78 miles/126 kilometers

On the road at 7:00 a.m., although later than usual, it was barely light at that time due to the central time zone being another hour earlier.

It was a beautiful morning, as the sun rose from the east. Lots of wide-open spaces and nothing in sight for miles. Nothing better than being away from the traffic on the interstate.

Highway 90 runs parallel to a train track, and to add to the scenery, freight trains roll by every now and again. I even got a couple of horn blasts from an engine driver for encouragement. It was one long lonely road today that kept disappearing into the sky. Wide-open prairies that ran up to desolate mountains all around.

There were a couple of small towns along the way that were pretty much ghost towns with no gas (petrol) stations or stores for 77 miles.

Just out of Valentine, in the middle of nowhere, is a Prada shop built in 2005 as "pop architecture land art." The shop is fully stocked with bags and shoes – seemed like a waste. Weird! Go check it out here: http://en.wikipedia.org/wiki/Prada_Marfa.

West Texas looked like the Australian outback. There were no kangaroos but plenty of antelope standing by the road, just watching me go by.

I arrived in Marfa at 2:30 p.m., a pleasant little town founded in the 1880s as a railroad water stop. It was also part of the mail route from San Antonio to San Diego.

The town of Marfa has been the backdrop for a bunch of movies, including *Giant*, starring James Dean, and *St. Elmo's Fire*. The town is famous for the Marfa Lights that appear at night in various colors as they move about the sky (featured on *Unsolved Mysteries* and in an episode of *King of the Hill*). The town of Marfa also holds a film festival each year. I plan to make it back for that at some point in the future.

Stats for the Day:

Distance – 78 miles/126 kilometers
Ride time – 6 hours
Average speed – 12.89 mph/20.7 kph
Elevation – 4,714 ft

The Route:

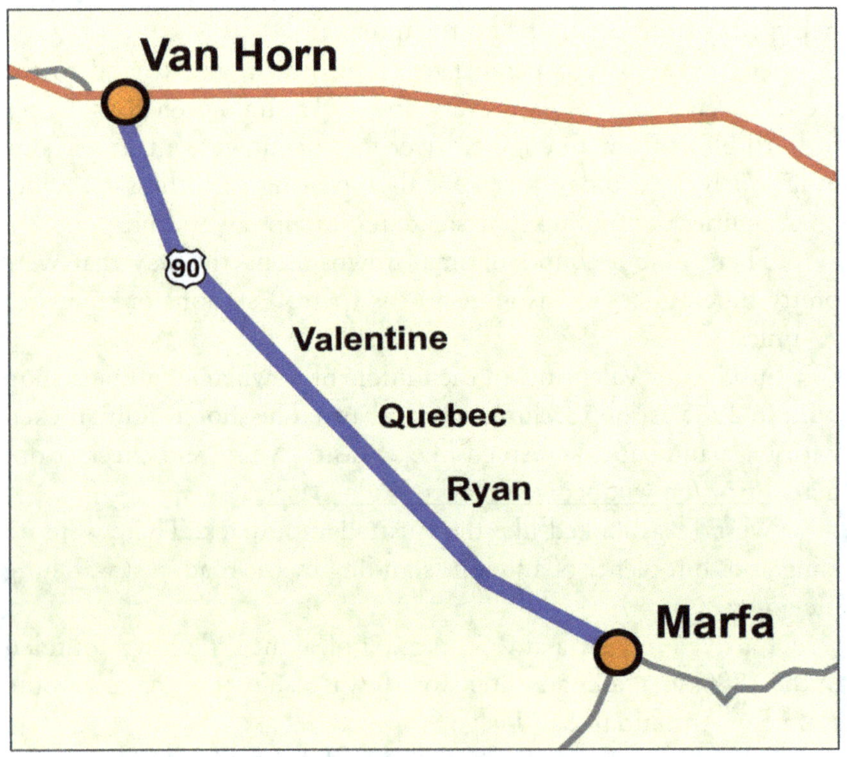

From Van Horn to Marfa, Texas.

Pictures of the Day:

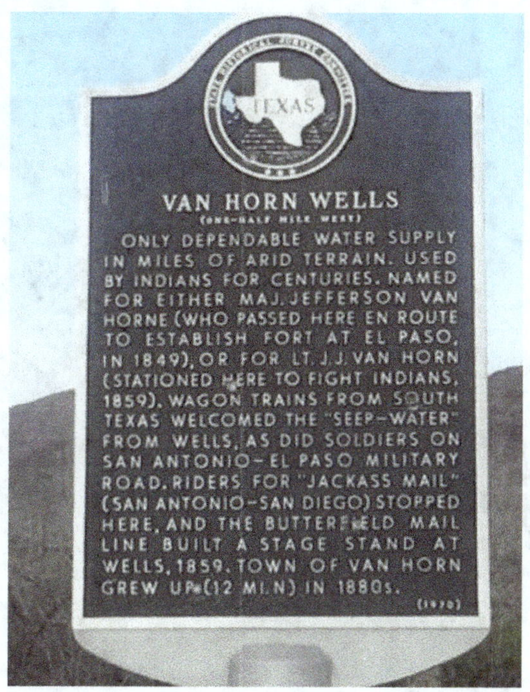

I couldn't see any water or Indians.

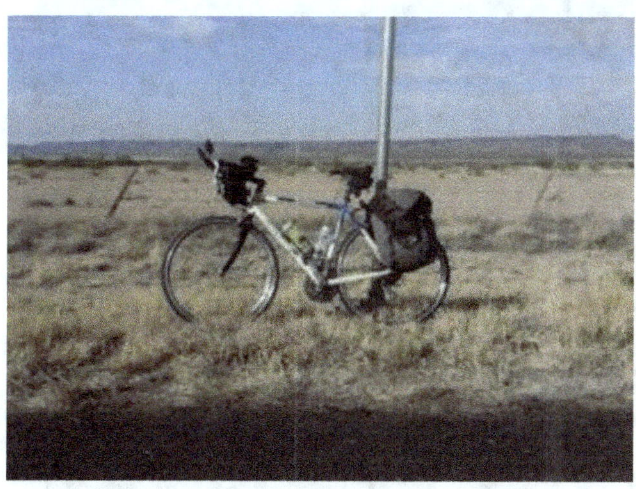

Quiet lunch stop in the middle of nowhere.

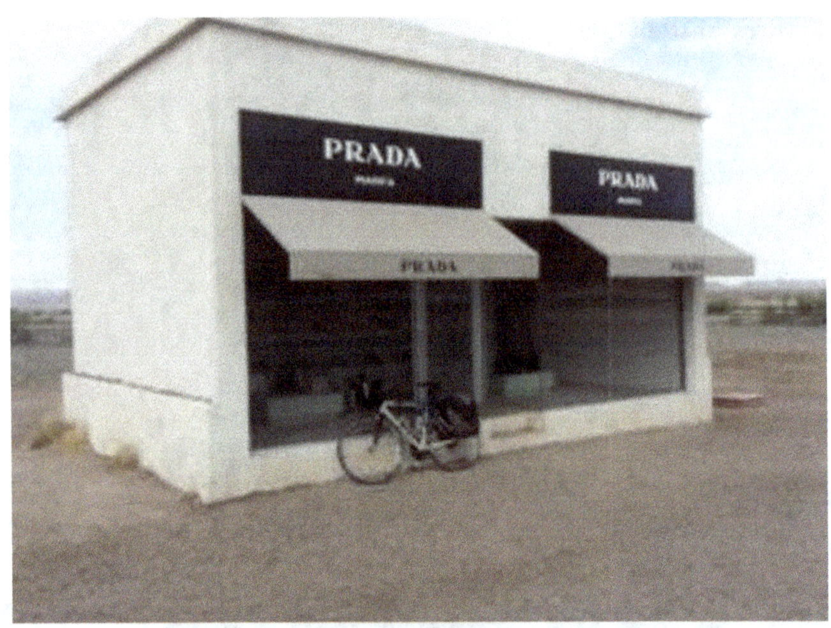

Prada art project.

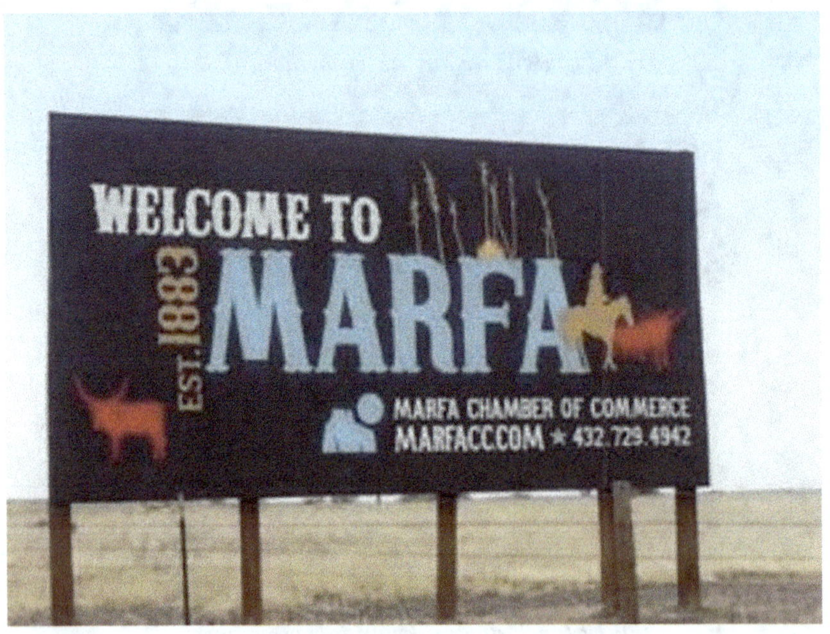

Quite an interesting little town.

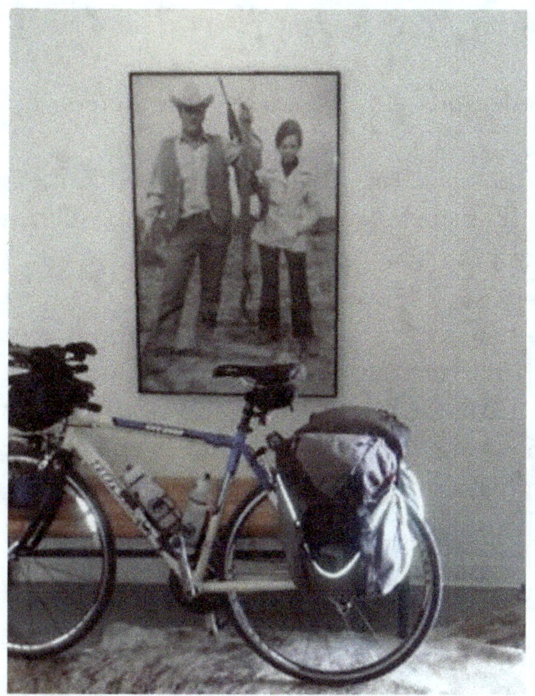

Hotel room painted floor with cowhides and cool picture.

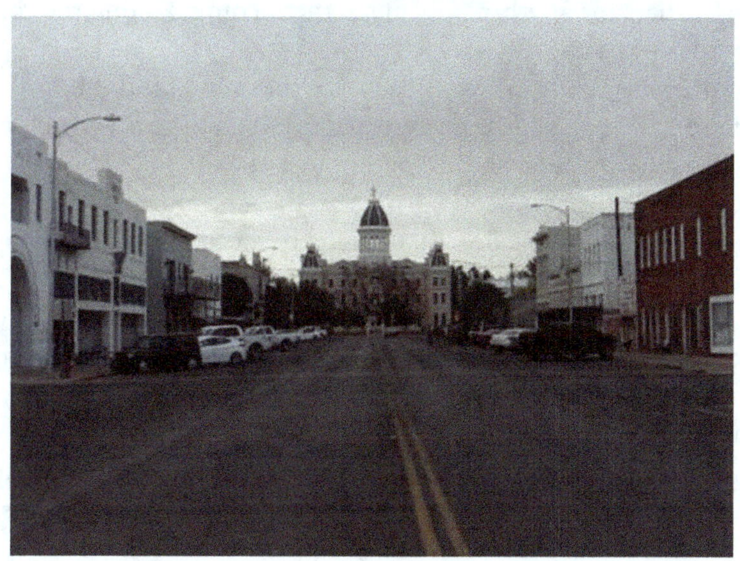

Downtown Marfa.

Day 4: Sunday, May 5, 2013

Marfa to Sanderson – 115 miles/185 kilometers

I was on the road at 6:45 a.m. today and looking forward to a downhill run. The sun appeared from behind the Chinati Mountains, filling the sky from orange to dark blue, but again, there was the relentless wind.

Highway 90 is a fairly good road with a wide shoulder, not too much traffic, and very few trucks. I've passed through five counties and one can tell because of the various postings at the side of the road (if you are watching) or the change in road surfaces. Jeff Davis County has the smoothest road surface finish of all, almost like the interstate. The others went low budget – plenty of gravel and not much tar.

At Paisano Pass, just out of Marfa, the elevation is over 5,000 feet and the temperature around 40°F. This was the highest point of the ride.

I arrived in Alpine around 9:00 a.m. and had a great breakfast at Penny's Diner with the local cowboys. They never seem to take off those big hats for anything. I can see them coming along the road in their trucks wearing *the hat*.

After breakfast, it was back to the wind and 90 miles to Sanderson. The rest of the day was pretty much head down and mind games to pass the next six and half hours.

So here's what I worked out: at the optimum speed of 16.5 mph, any aches and pains that might be occurring just disappear. Anything under that speed, everything hurts!

The good thing about the wind was that I was getting to stop at more historical markers and brush up on the local history. Some of the markers were quite interesting with names of well-known people from that time.

I passed through the small town of Marathon, which clearly outlined the day – marathon. I'm past the halfway mark for this ride at 324 miles completed and only 280 miles to San Antonio.

Stats for the Day:

Distance – 115 miles/185 kilometers
Ride time – 9 hours
Average speed – 12.8 mph/20.6 kph
Elevation – 2,760 ft

The Route:

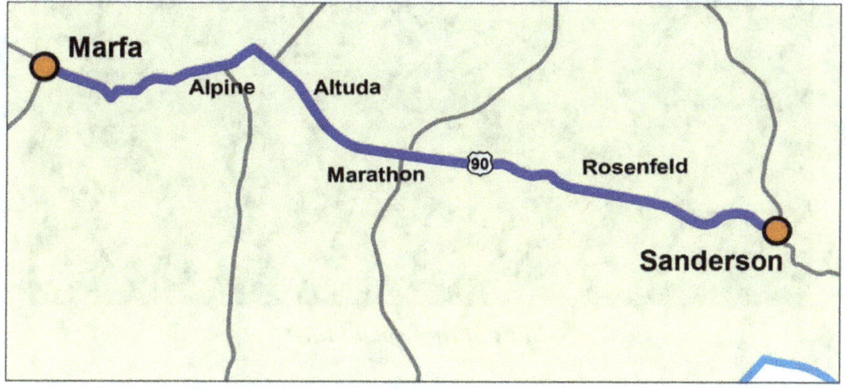

From Marfa to Sanderson, Texas.

This could be helpful info: I've also worked out my favorite post workout sports drink. Something that helps refresh and revive after nine and a half hours ride – an icy cold Corona! So cold that as you pour it from the bottle into a glass, icicles form in the beverage. Happy Cinco de Mayo.

Pictures of the Day:

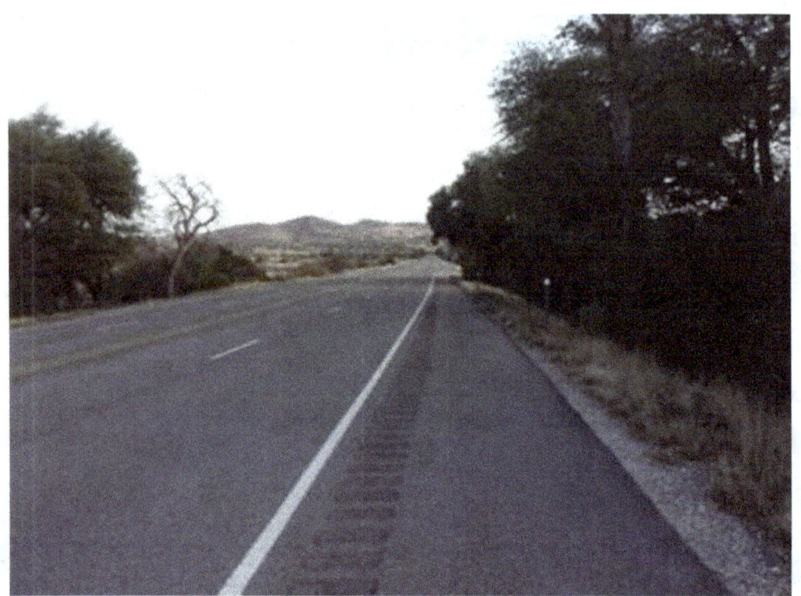

Start of the "downhill."

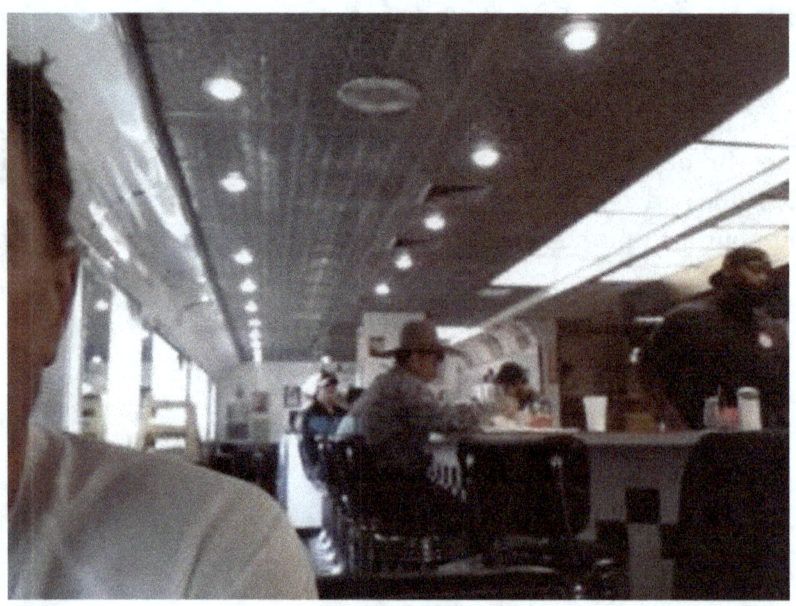

Texas diner – big hats are all the go.

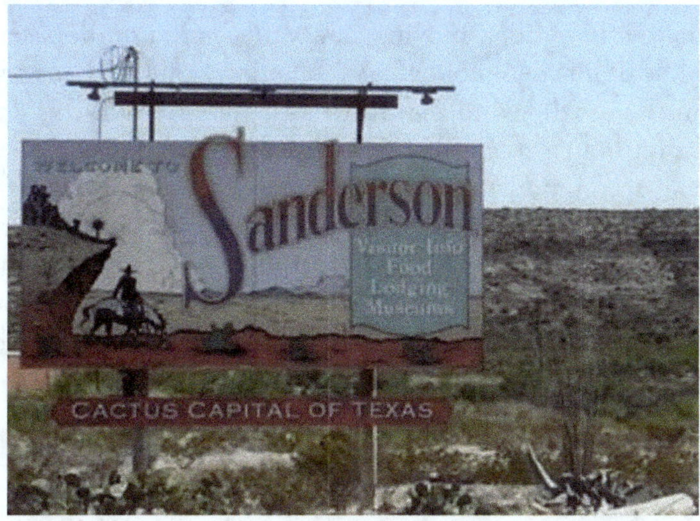

Welcome to the Cactus Capital of Texas – Sanderson.

Day 5: Monday, May 6, 2013

Sanderson to Comstock – 90 miles/145 kilometers

I spent the night with a chair against the hotel door and my bike light on the night stand – just in case. These small towns don't seem to get much traffic. Their heydays are long gone. Interstate 10 is an easier road to travel. Young people have moved to big cities for work, leaving their generational homes behind. This lack of economy was reflected in the quality of some of the hotels and the age of their rooms. When I checked in last night, there was no hot water, but *we* eventually got it working.

This riding is a *job*, so I was on the road at 6:45 a.m. today. There was no continental breakfast at the hotel, but the service station near the hotel was open. So I grabbed a plastic bagged cheese Danish and a coffee. Then I stood around the side of the building with the cats, out of the wind to enjoy.

Reading the historical plaque about a train robber, a sidekick of Butch Cassidy and the Sundance Kid, I think about what it must have been like to cross this country on horse or stagecoach. My mind wanders to a lone rider, moving across the tundra on horseback, in the middle of nowhere, following a long dusty trail. No one around, no sound – just the wind that races past my ears. Will this day end with a camp out or in a town? What will that town offer – food, water and accommodations?

It was a long grind today with the headwind, a constant companion stealing every downhill opportunity for any momentum or speed. I went quicker uphill as the road was a little more protected from the wind, with speeds around 6–12 mph. On the crest, the full force of the southeasterly wind dropped my bike speed back to 8–10 mph. This was reflected in my average speed for the day at 10.28 miles per hour. To compare, on the first 900 miles of my ride from San Diego to El Paso, I averaged 15.5 miles per hour.

I didn't stop in Dryden, as there didn't seem to be much going on. So I pushed on another 40 miles to Langtry, the town famous for Judge Roy Bean. Looks like he hung quite a few people, as the town had about eight residents. The Langtry Museum was about a mile off the highway and I really didn't need an extra two miles today.

There was a small gas station at the main intersection. There was no one around or any other stores. It seemed like there was some movement inside that gas station. What a surprise! There was a small kitchen that made a great burrito lunch. I enjoyed lunch with what I reckon was half the town – the cook, the server, the judge (he could have passed for Judge Roy Bean), and a guy who turned up on an ATV, drinking a beer. We all sat around the one table in the place and discussed long distance cycling, the weather, and the current depth of the Rio Grande.

The highway followed the Rio Grande (Big River) which marks the border between the US and Mexico. Although I didn't see much traffic, I'm sure the border patrol watched me all day with all their surveillance equipment, maybe taking bets on when or *if* I would make it into Comstock. I can visualize them in a control room somewhere, watching their monitors through the day. "What's the lone biker up to?" one of them yells out. Then they're all cheering and high-fiving when I make it into Comstock after nine hours on the road.

The Comstock Motel was a shock after the last few nights. It had just been remodeled. I could live in this hotel, at least for two nights anyway. As I pulled up to the hotel, the guy working the front desk had his Ford F250 backed up to the office door with a barbeque on the tailgate cooking a steak. It smelled great!

There's probably an app already for this, but I made up a new game called Line Rider. It involves keeping your tires on the three-inch white line that separates the roadway from the shoulder. It's difficult to ride the thin line, but it's smooth with a buildup of white paint. On one side of the line you have the shoulder – generally rough, covered in rocks, blown truck tires, nails, screws, bolts, glass, and dead animals, but generally safe. On the other side, you have the clean roadway that is smoothed out from all the heavy traffic but can be dangerous for cyclists. Just concentrate and keep an eye on the rear view mirror for traffic. Note: Keep away from the white line when it's wet; they become extremely slippery.

Stats for the Day:

Distance – 90 miles/145 kilometers
Ride time – 8 hours 20 minutes
Average speed – 10.28 mph/16.5 kph
Elevation – 1,580 ft

The Route:

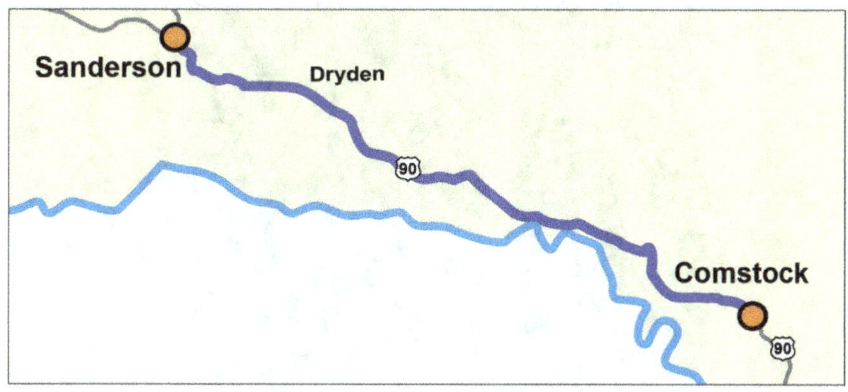

From Sanderson to Comstock, Texas.

Pictures of the Day:

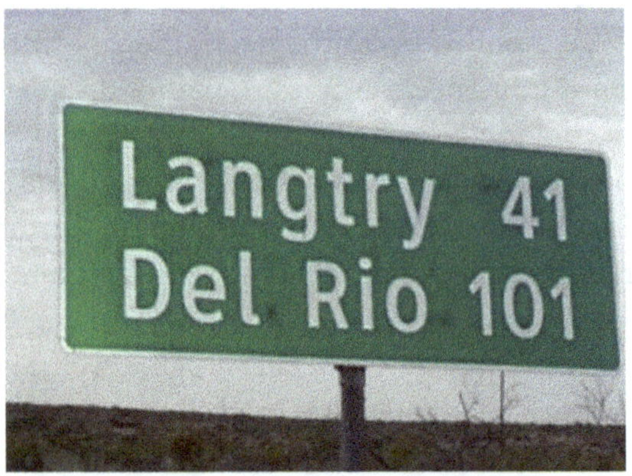

That's okay. It's only 101 miles!

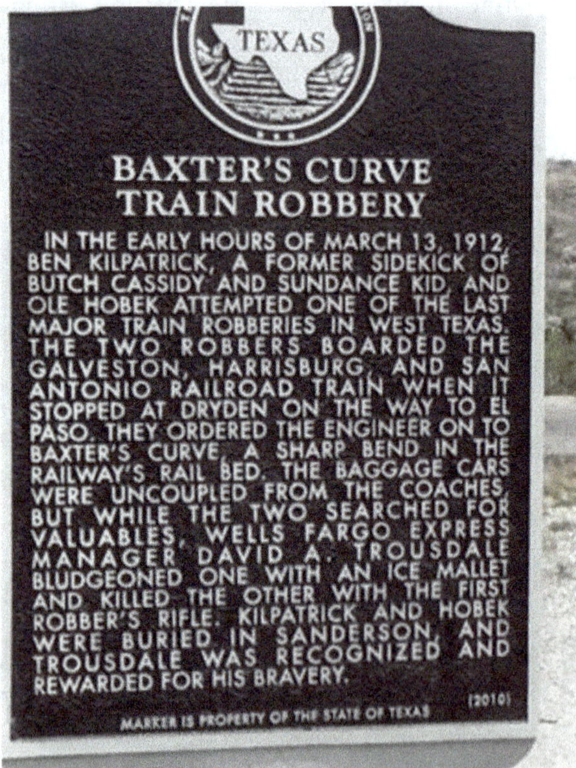

Great story. Butch Cassidy and the Sundance Kid.

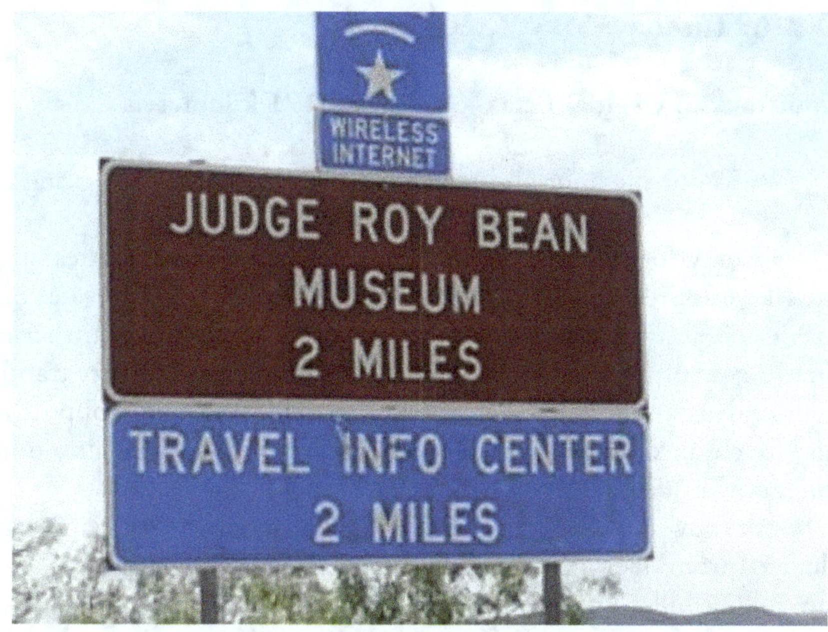

Wireless Internet okay, but what about food and water?

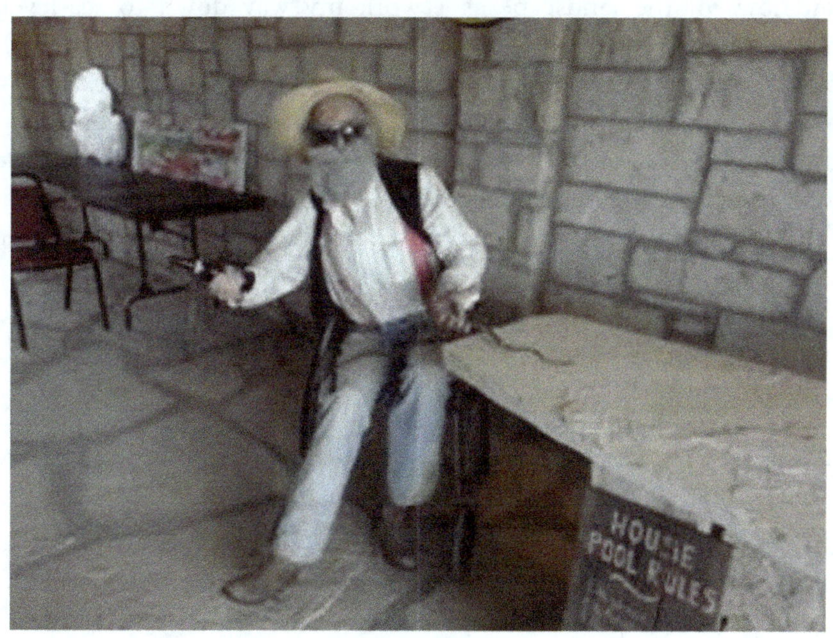

At the judge's café.

Day 6: Tuesday, May 7, 2013

Comstock to Uvalde, Texas – 106 miles/171 kilometers

I was out the door and ready for battle at 6:35 a.m. – bring it on!

Twenty-four miles along is Amistad Lake Recreation Area and the lake was probably 10 percent full. Maybe they sent the water on to Mexico, just the other side of the dam wall. Eight miles further is Del Rio, a surprisingly big town where I encounter my first traffic light in five days. Of course, I stop on red. This was a good opportunity for a quick breakfast, then onto Bracketville, another thirty odd miles down the road.

I'm now in the Texas Hill Country and the landscape has changed from open desert with mountain ranges to green trees and low rolling hills. This is really deer/antelope hunting country with feeders and towers everywhere and game wardens.

The roads are like one big, long snake lying across the highs and lows of the landscape as I work my way down to sea-level. Surprisingly, I haven't seen any snakes on this leg of the journey (yet), but everyone I meet talks about how *big* the snakes are in Texas.

Coming into Brackettville was a good old Texas barbeque right there on the side of the road. Time for some pulled pork tacos. Life looks pretty simple for these ladies running the barbeque – no shop front, just a big barbeque trailer and some tables and chairs in the shade of a large tree. No cash register and cash only.

I took advantage of the wind today. Although this devil wind had been stealing all my momentum, it did help keep me cool while riding. Around 2:00 p.m., the temperature was at 103°F.

One of my concerns on this trip, and especially over the last couple of days, has been riding solo so close to the Mexican border. I'm way past that area of concern now, and the border patrol is doing their job. They were *everywhere*. Just across the US border is Ciudad Acuna / Del Rio. This is another of the illegal drug routes into the United States from these border towns.

I arrived in Uvalde around 4:30 p.m. Over the last six days, I have ridden this bike 520 miles and logged 43 hours in the saddle. I've met many characters along the way and have seen a lot of the beautiful west Texas countryside. I've also passed the halfway point of my adventurous plan to ride across America. I only have 1,200 miles now until I finish on the Atlantic Ocean in Florida.

Tomorrow I have 90 miles into San Antonio and my final destination for this trip. As a tribute to all the people mentioned on the historical markers along my Texas ride, and my battle against the headwinds, I'm planning on finishing this ride at the Alamo in downtown San Antonio, the most famous Texas tourist attraction whose history is ingrained in the great state of Texas. Check it out: http://en.wikipedia.org/wiki/Battle_of_the_Alamo.

Stats for the Day:

Distance – 106 miles/171 kilometers
Ride time – 8 hours 50 minutes
Average speed – 11.94 mph/19.21 kph
Elevation – 862 ft

The Route:

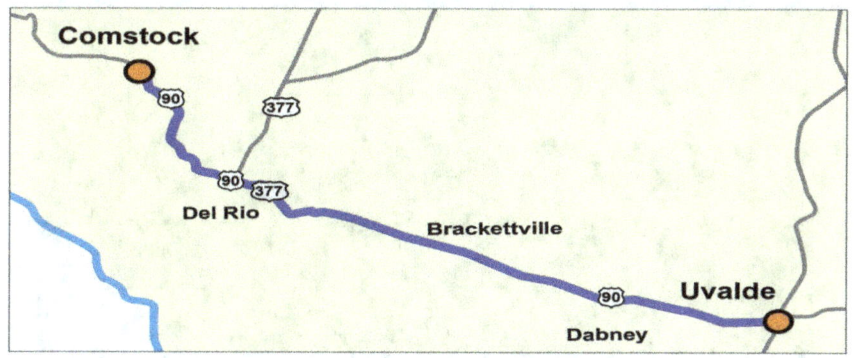

From Comstock to Uvalde, Texas.

Pictures of the Day:

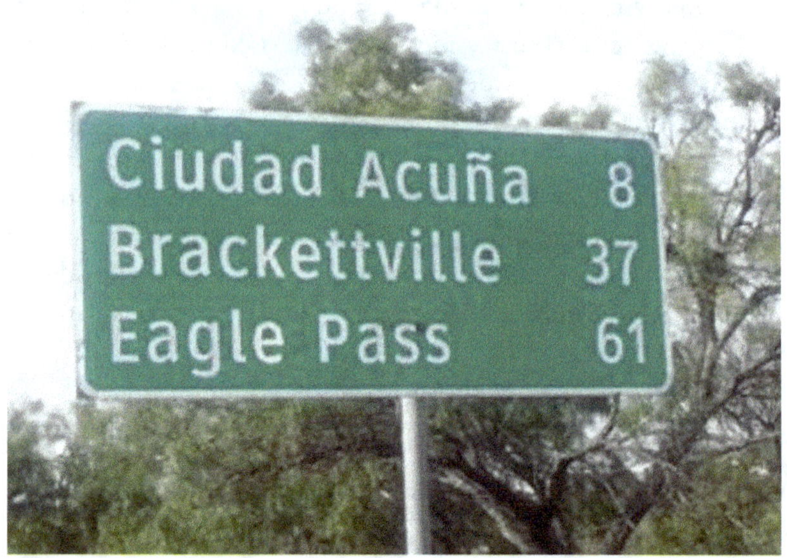

Close to Mexico again – Ciudad Acuna, Mexico

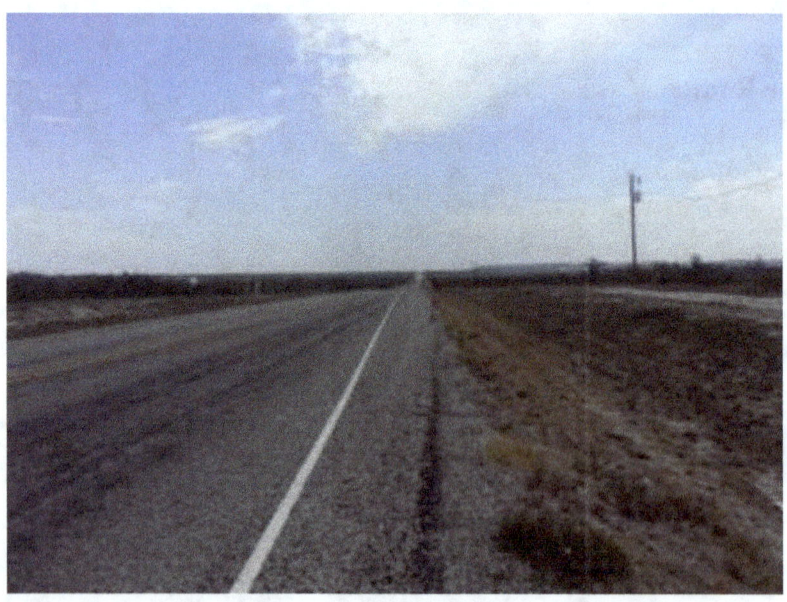

That's a long straight road to San Antonio.

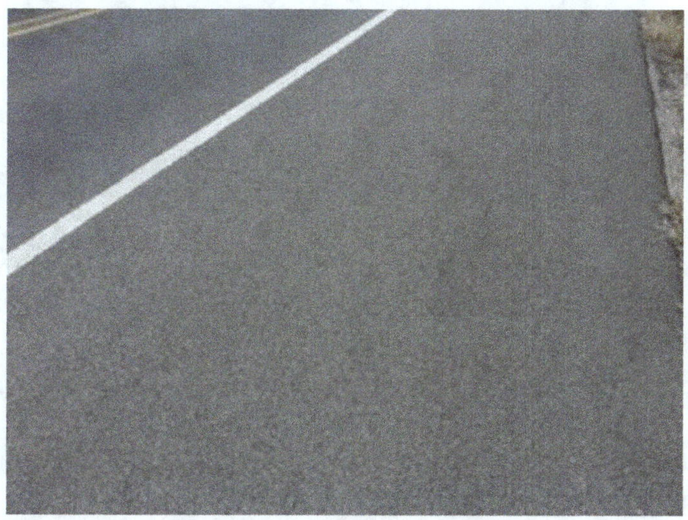

Bicyclist's dream – smooth, clean, wide shoulder and easy on the knees.

Day 7: Wednesday, May 8, 2013

Uvalde to San Antonio – 100 miles/161 kilometers

I was really in the mood for an Italian feed, so last night the closest place to the hotel was the Pizza Hut in Uvalde. And it was awesome. A thin-crust with pepperoni and black olives.

Although the hotel was great, I was on the road early today. I always feel good on the last day of the trip and ready to get this last section done. As a bonus today, I have a mate who is meeting me on the outskirts of San Antonio and riding with me as a tour guide for the San Antonio Missions.

There are four missions we will be touring today on our way to the Alamo. The missions were built in the early 1700s by the Spanish to convert Native Americans to Christianity, while helping to settle the region under Spanish rule.

The missions are located on either side of the banks along the San Antonio River. Along the river there is a nice bike path most of the way. We did, however, have to take a couple of really busy highways before we got to the sanctuary of the bike path.

I met Dan about forty miles from San Antonio and he was ready to ride. His bike was clean and shiny. Dan was decked out in all the gear, his legs were fresh, and he was not carrying any luggage.

We took a break at the first mission (Mission Espada) and toured the building and the grounds. Then we went on to Mission San Juan and Mission San Jose. Finally, we were at the last – Mission Conception, which was really nice. I have to say the missions were very cool, but my mind was on getting to the Alamo, my hotel, and a hot shower.

On the busy streets of downtown San Antonio, the Alamo finally appears. It is an awesome site! I am thankful to be here safely. Dan and Bob are keen to meet up for a margarita and toast my ride. Who am I to say no to an offer like that?

Tonight, Sara flew in from Phoenix, so it was dinner on the River Walk in downtown San Antonio. We are staying at the famous Mengar Hotel, which has hosted many United States Presidents and other dignitaries from around the world.

Stats for the Day:

Distance – 100 miles/161 kilometers
Ride time – 7 hours 50 minutes
Average speed – 12.9 mph/20.8 kph
Elevation – 772 ft

The Route:

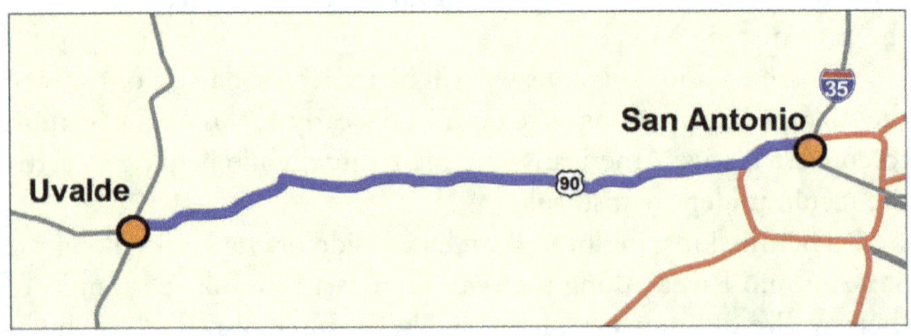

From Uvalde to San Antonio.

Pictures of the Day:

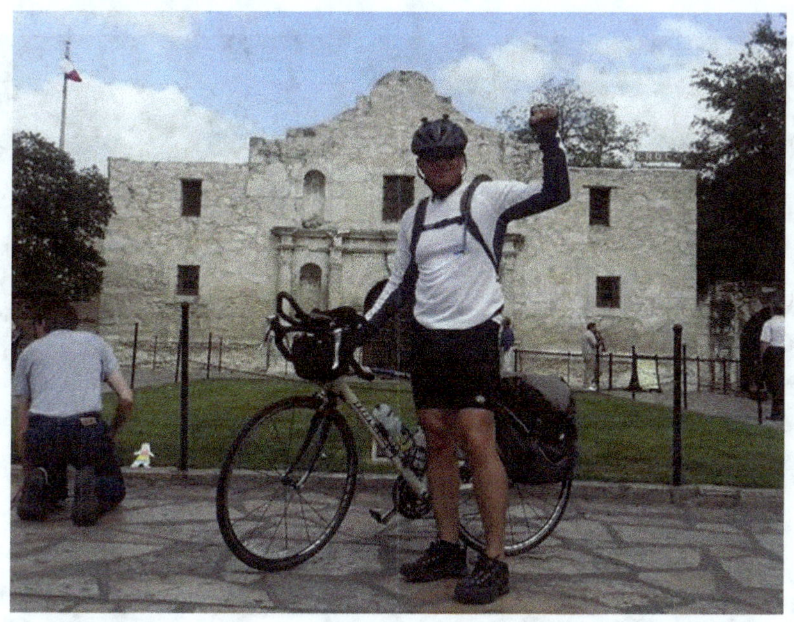

Big finish at the Alamo, San Antonio, with Flat Stanley photo bombing.

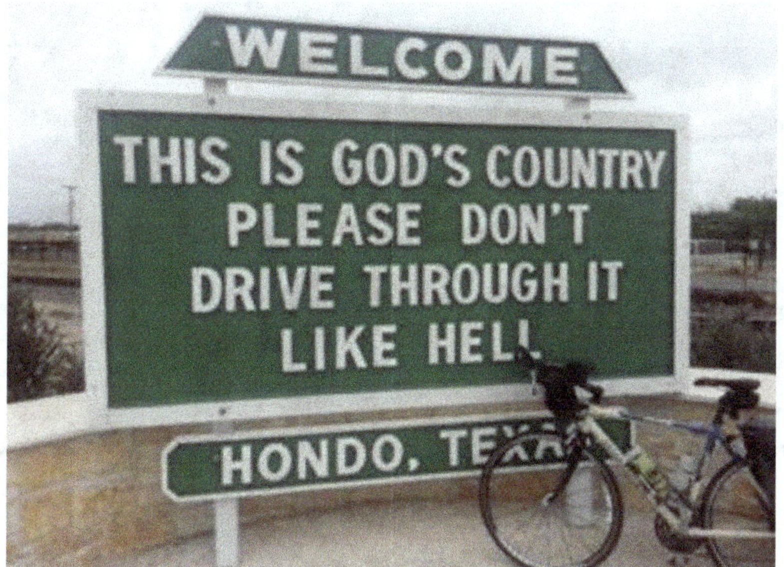

That's telling them.

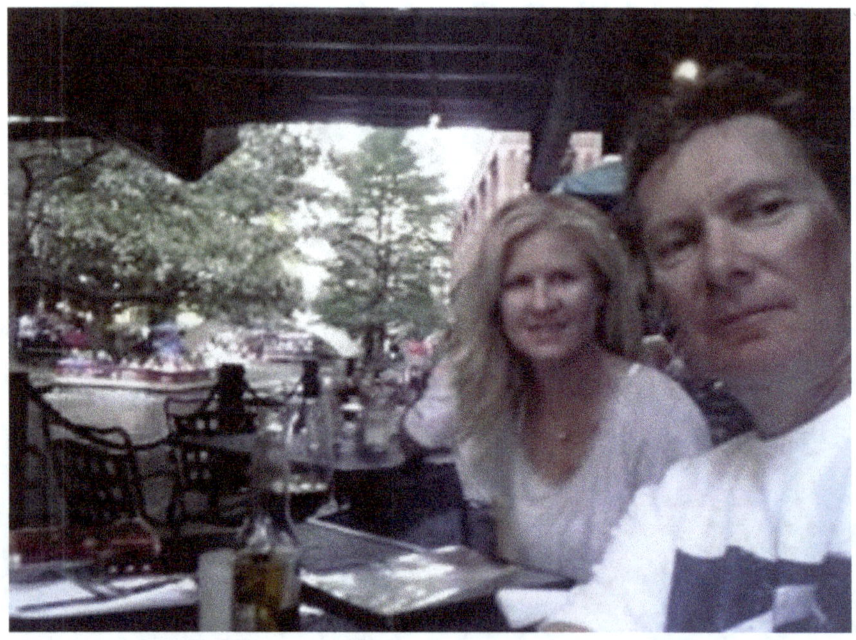

A great dinner with Sara on the Riverwalk in San Antonio.

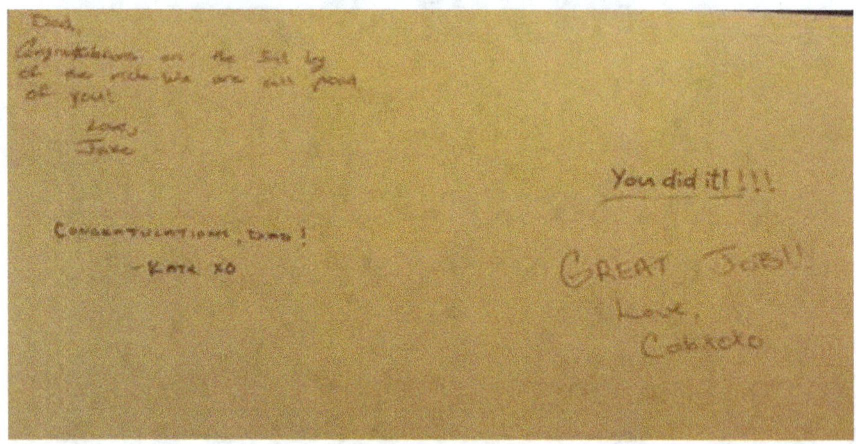

Family card.

Planning for my ride.

El Paso to San Antonio

mph 15

Date	Day		Daily Miles	Daily Kms	Miles Between	Miles Accum.	Time	Rain	High-Low	Wind	Shane's Notes - October 16, 2012
Thurs - 5/2	1 El Paso	Fort Hancock	54	87	50		4.3	0%	70-49	E 22	Forthancockmotel.com
Fri - 5/3	2 Fort Hancock	Serria Blanca			40	90		0%	76-49	SSE 12	10 miles of interstate
	Serria Blanca	Allagmore			22	112					Interstate 10
	Allagmore	Van Horn	77	124	11	123	6.3				Interstate 10
Sat - 5/4	3 Van Horn	Lobo			17	140		0%	81-54	SW 21	Pilot gas station turn off I10
	Lobo	Valentine			26	166					Small small town - nothing
	Valentine	Marfa	78	126	35	201	6.0				Plan on bringing Lunch & Water
Sun - 5/5	4 Marfa	Alpine #			26	227		10%	83-48	SSW 12	Plenty of food and accommodation - breakfas
	Alpine	Altuda			16	243					Ramda Hampton Inn plenty of stuff - bigger th
	Altuda	Marathon #			15	258					appears to be nothing here ... Nothing
	Marathon	Sanderson	115	185	55	313	9.0				Marathon Hotel, coffee place gage hotel looks
Mon - 5/6	5 Sanderson	Dryden			21	334		20%	85-59	ESE 14	2 hotels coming into town. Stripes gas station
	Dryden	Langtry			40	374					little grocery store - no accoms no gas station
	Langtry	Comstock	90	145	29	403	8.2				Nothing but a turn off Hwy 90. - http://www.la
Tue - 5/7	6 Comstock	Amistad Lake			24	427		10%	91-68	SE 11	Coming in RV park with Cabins - this looks OK
	Amistad Lake	Los Campos			4	431					Amistad lake resort hotel, gas station - look g
	Los Campos	Del Rio			4	435					Los Campos
	Del Rio	Brackettville			31	466					La Quinta $65 / Hampton, Walmart big town
	Brackettville	Cline			21	487					ft clark springs motel/rv/restaurant, subway,
	Cline	Uvalde	105	169	19	506	9.0				Nothing in Cline
Wed - 5/8	7 Uvalde	Knippa			10	516		10%	90-67	SE 10	Quality Inn, big town
	Knippa	Sabinal			11	517					Knippa
	Sabinal	D'Hanis			12	528					gas x 2, Ogden's Motor Inn, Twin Oaks Motel
	D'Hanis	Hondo			9	537					D'Hanis
	Hondo	Castroville			17	554					large town, Executive Inn
	Castroville	The Alamos SAT	100	161	28	582	7.5	10%	87-65	SE 11	Castroville
				619			50				

CHAPTER 5

San Antonio, Texas to New Orleans, Louisiana September 20–26, 2014

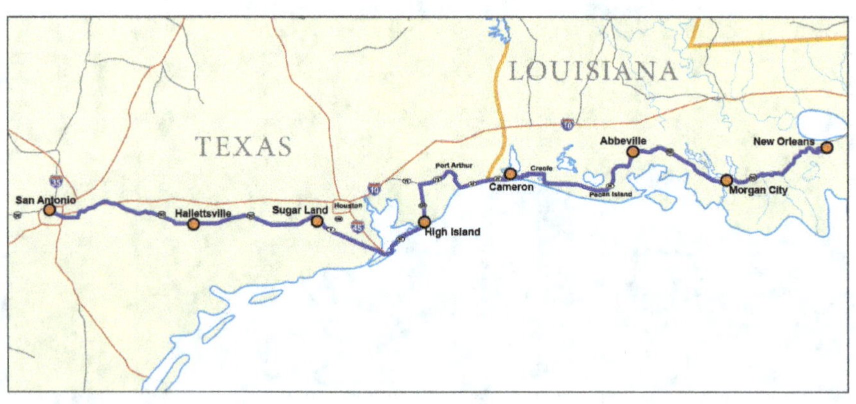

Total distance – 653 miles/1052 kilometers
Number of days – 7 days
Average speed – 13.4 mph/21.6 kph
Total saddle time – 48 hours

Day 1: Saturday, September 20, 2014

San Antonio to Hallettsville, Texas – 102.80 miles/165 kilometers

That was a good first day . . . riding through the Texas Hill Country, and tonight I'm in Hallettsville, the "City of Hospitality" (the sign indicated on the way in). I kicked off the day near the San Antonio airport this morning around 5:40 a.m. and arrived into Hallettsville around 2:30 p.m., just over 100 miles. There is lots of humidity with a few showers this morning, then sunny this afternoon. Temperatures are hovering around 75 F early on, then 90 F, with that familiar cooling headwind from the east at about 10–15 mph.

The morning section was back to the chip seal shoulder and the afternoon through Gonzales County paying the extra for a pavement finish. It was so smooth that I could feel even the smallest loose stone as I cruised along. I think I've worked this out (why the road composition is different in each county): higher gas (petrol) prices provide extra taxes and that equals better roads.

It was meant to be a 72-miler today, but the hotel that I wanted to stay in at Shiner, Texas, was booked out. So I pushed on. The Town of Shiner is the home of one of my favorite beers and the Spoetzl Brewery, the oldest independent brewery in Texas. The brewery is most well known for producing Shiner Bock, a dark German/Czech-style beer. My mate, Eddie, who lives up in the Texas panhandle, put me on to it a few years back, and I've since had a few kegs of this through my kegorator.

It was a little eerie peddling in the dark so early today. People were pulling their roller bags with no airport or hotels in sight. Once I was clear of the city and it became daylight, there were some really nice little towns along the way. Saturday must be the designated day for cutting grass; every town I passed through had people out driving their ride on mower. There's nothing better than the smell of fresh cut grass. Going through these towns would make a great ride for a motorcycle or convertible!

I've driven Interstate 10 Highway many times between San Antonio and Houston for business, coming across the usual roadside offering that is all the same stuff. The back roads on the other hand, offer up a variety of local diners, grocery stores, and specialty shops. Today I was on Highway 90, heading east. This back road alternative is something I will ponder more while riding tomorrow.

The first day of these rides are always tough. I'm getting settled in, making sure my gear is all secure and set. As I ride, I think of things, and the smallest issue (that really means nothing) can become a huge mental distraction until I stop and fix it or simply adjust something. Then the mind moves on to the next possible problem. As the day progresses, the head finally clears of all the Google clutter and I become focused on the ride and the positives, "Today's ride I've completed 16 percent of this week's ride to New Orleans!"

If you haven't seen an armadillo before, see the picture below. Looked like he was sleeping.

I saw a really cool old car today, somewhere near Shiner, and had to take a picture of it. If you know what make, model and year it is, please let me know.

Stats for the Day:

Distance travelled – 102.80 miles/165 kilometers
Average speed – 13.4 mph/21.56 kph
Time – 8 hours 41 minutes
Calories burned – 7,542

The Route:

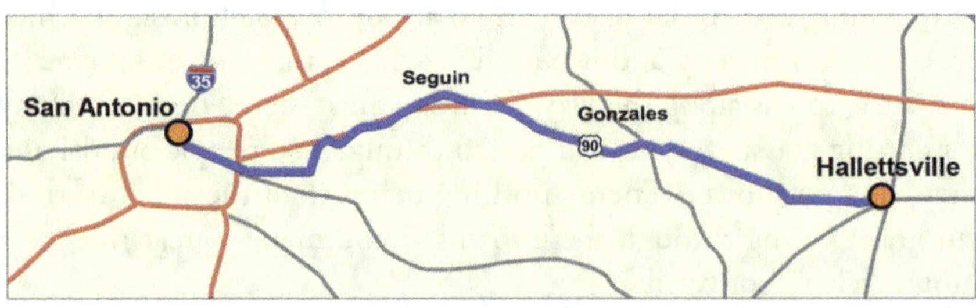

From San Antonio to Hallettsville, Texas.

Pictures of the Day:

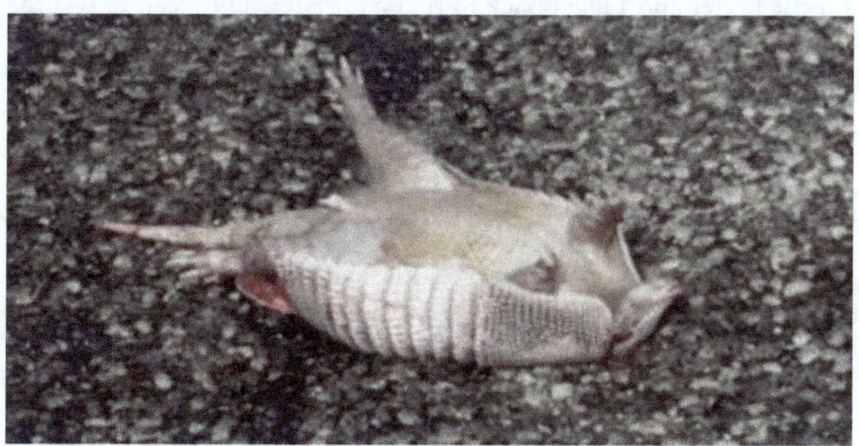

Upside-down armadillo

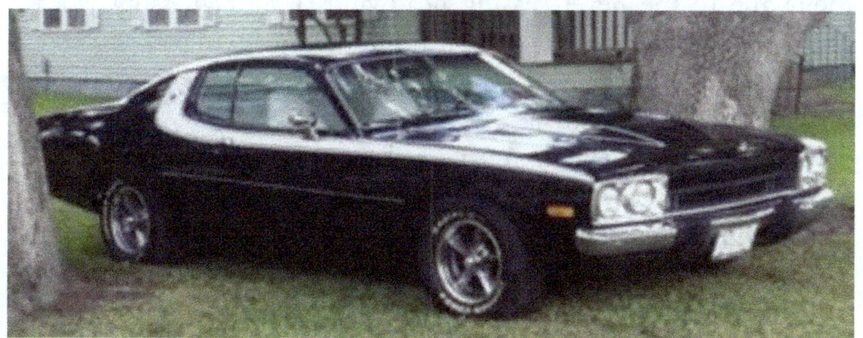

Mystery car that caught my eye this morning.

Day 2: Sunday, September 21, 2014

Hallettsville to Sugarland, Texas – 92 miles/148 kilometers

My body just realized today that we are doing that thing again. I grabbed a coffee and an apple, then out the door at 5:40 a.m. with an 83-mile (134-kilometer) ride to Sugerland, just outside Houston, Texas. I made a wrong turn toward the end and added an extra nine miles to the trip. It was my fault, not concentrating, but it turned out for the better and I'll get back to that a bit later. The weather was the same as yesterday, but no rain, less humidity, and the same headwind directly from the east. Before sunrise, the air is still and I can feel the increased speed of the bike over yesterday's ride. Then as the sun rises, along comes the wind.

I'm in the Hill Country for the first 40 miles today, and there are beautiful woodlands on either side of the road. In a clearing just on daylight, I go past three large whitetail deer. They are standing in the mist. They turn and run off, with only the whites of their tails visible.

I can hear the weekend hunters out shooting. It's Texas, after all. I can smell their campfires and am thinking that they are having coffee or cooking bacon and eggs. That sounds really good about now!

When it comes to dead animals, I can smell them before I see them due to the never-ceasing headwind. I start guessing what it could be – armadillo, badger, bird, rabbit, turtle, snake, or deer? It doesn't turn out to be any of these, but a dog, quite large, and a bad omen for the rest of the day.

I've had a few encounters with dogs since San Diego, mainly in the smaller rural communities. It seems like the more run-down the house, the crazier the dogs. The dead dog from earlier put the curse on me as I had three close calls later in the day.

Here's how it goes down. They are usually lying around the yard listening to the cars and trucks go by, then they hear something different – my bike coming. I hear them barking. We see each other at the same time, our eyes lock, and the race is now on. None of them caught me today, but I was thinking about what I would do if they did:

1. Yell at the dog to back off.
2. If this doesn't work, get off the bike and use it as my primary line of defense.
3. Pull out the pepper spray and blast away.
4. If this doesn't work, it's time to bring out my knife.

No different to a bear, mountain lion, or misguided encounter with a human. Well, I think that's what I'd do.

After Eagle Lake, the Hill Country is behind me and I'm pretty much at sea level. There are lots of paddocks full of cotton and other produce lined by long, flat, straight roads. I see an overpass in the distance, maybe four or five miles ahead, a good spot to take a break from the sun. I start really looking forward to it and plan what snack I'll eat. It takes *forever* to get there! Then a road sign appears: "Texas Department of Criminal Justice – Parole Office." The shade got the better of me and I took a five-minute break while constantly on watch. It's Sunday and things are quiet, although there are people working. Most of these towns have a population between seven hundred and three thousand people. Soon, I'm in Rosenburg and surprised to see the population jump to thirty-five thousand, definitely getting close to a major city – Houston is about 30 miles east of here.

I'm staying at the Best Western, the most upscale hotel until I get into New Orleans. The accommodations along the beach route are not that well advertised or rated. I called ahead for accommodations tomorrow at the Gulf Beach Motel/Restaurant in High Island. The lady on the phone quoted me $52 for the night. I offered my credit card to secure the room, and she said in her best Southern accent, "No need, *darling*. We'll see you tomorrow night!"

Back to the extra miles that I didn't need today . . . Coming along an access road to a freeway, there's a turtle trying to navigate up the curb to get back to the grass and mud. He had fallen back to the concrete, ending up on his back in the hot sun. I'm about one hundred yards past him. I pull up, turn around, and head back through the oncoming traffic to rescue the little guy. Back to the grass, you! I gave him a cold shower with the remaining water that I was carrying, my good deed for the day.

I was looking forward to getting to Galveston, Texas, tomorrow and seeing all that water along the Gulf of Mexico.

Stats for the Day:

Distance travelled – 92 miles/148 kilometers
Average speed – 13.1 mph/21.08 kph
Time – 6 hours 53 minutes
Calories burned – 5,554

The Route:

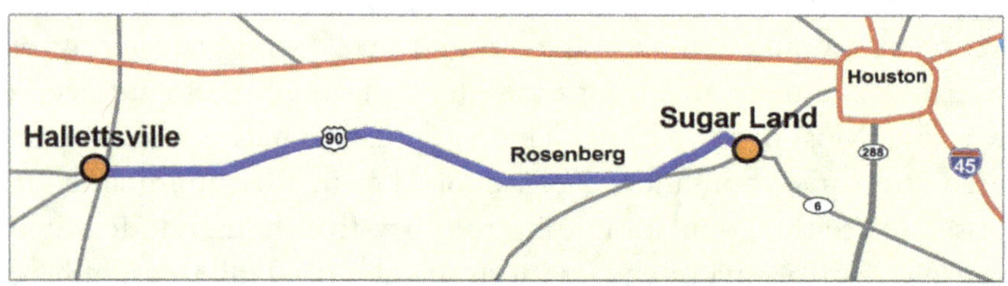

From Hallettsville to Sugarland, Texas.

Pictures of the Day:

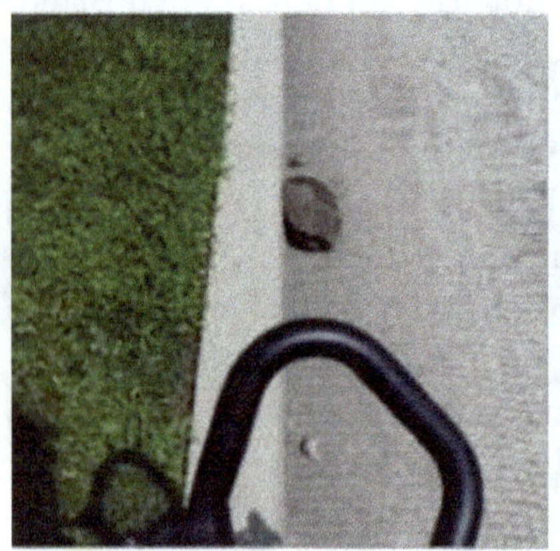
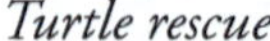

Turtle rescue

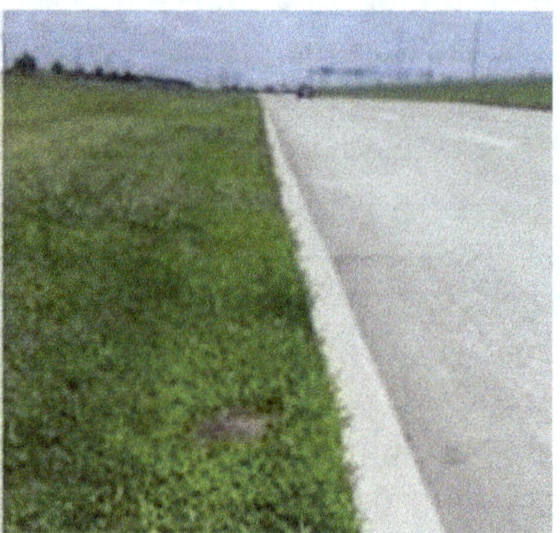

Safe in the grass

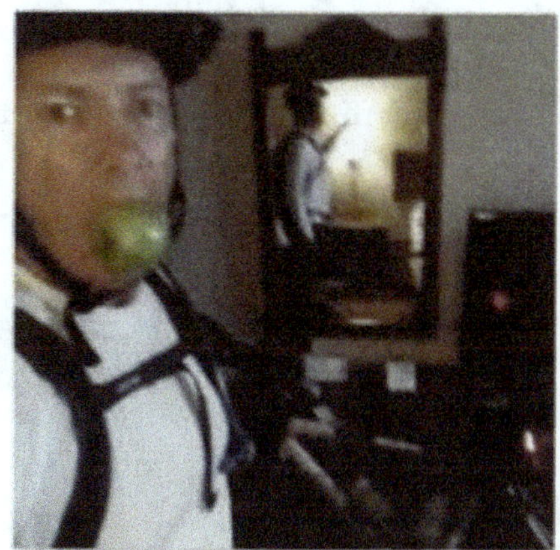

First breakfast

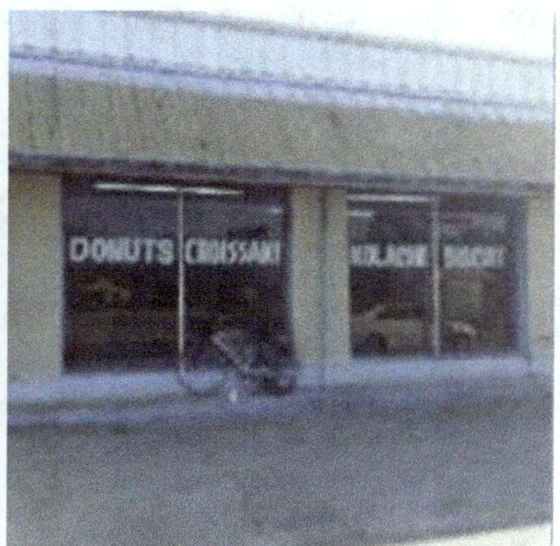

Second breakfast

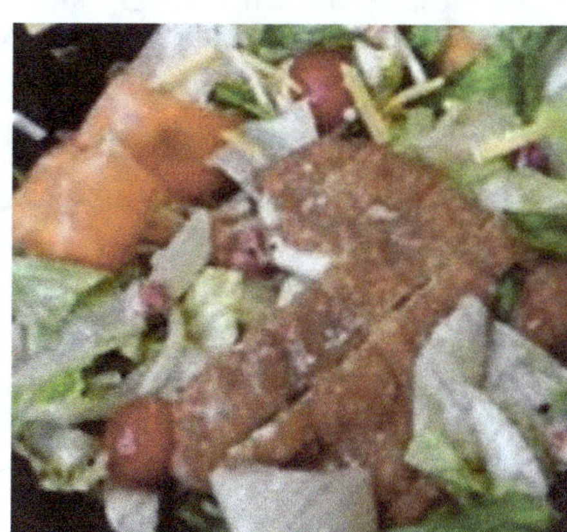

Lunch

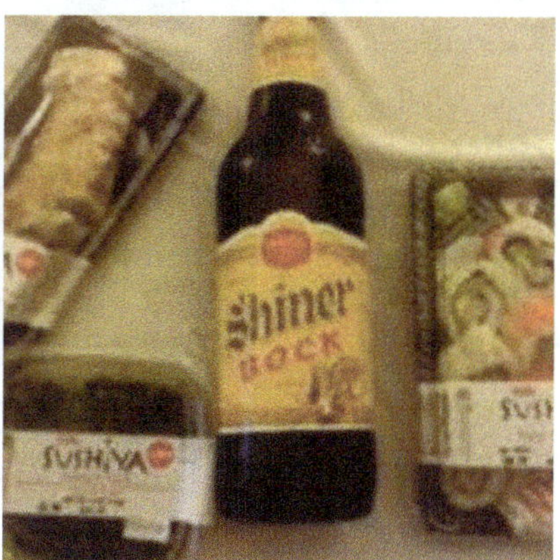

Dinner

Day 3: Monday, September 22, 2014

Sugarland to High Island, Texas – 97 miles/156 kilometers

I just can't lay here waiting for the alarm at 5:00 a.m. I may as well be out early and finish early. I was out the door at 4:20 a.m. with a coffee and banana.

I look like a well-lit Christmas tree moving along in the dark. I have the standard front and back headlight/taillights set up with a bunch of reflectors. And on my helmet, I have a white flashing light pointing forward and a red flashing light pointing backward. You really have to be doing a *long* text message not to see me!

About 7:20 a.m. in Algora, it's daylight and I'm moving nicely along Texas Highway 6, directly for Galveston. It's a really good road and part of the evacuation route when the hurricanes come roaring through the Gulf of Mexico. At 8:00 a.m., I'm in Hitchcock with almost 50 miles completed and ready for breakfast. Another 16 miles to the coast and I start to see bits of Galveston Bay on my right side. The smells are different now – diesel from the refineries, heavier air, and that fishy aroma. So I'm completely surrounded by water on either side of the road and ready to cross the causeway bridge on Interstate Highway 45. This is the only way across Galveston Bay, unless I go way west through Brazoria National Wildlife Refuge, adding an additional 77 miles to the route.

The only way to ride into this town is to have Glen Campbell playing "Galveston" – *I can hear your sea waves crashing . . .* Click here if you want to hear the tune: http://www.youtube.com/watch?v=tH-jWil-f3C8. Awesome bass guitar. Go on, turn it up.

I catch the ferry from Galveston Point to Bolivar Point, about a fifteen-minute boat ride across the mouth of the bay. There are boats coming and going and dolphins playing and jumping in front of the ferry. What a great day! I'm surrounded by water and I'm on a boat. This is a welcome change from the dry, southwestern deserts with so little water.

All the houses are elevated so they don't get washed away in the storms. I stop at a small shop for a snack. Pop's is the name of the store, and Pop is working the cash register. He tells me everything got wiped out in 2008 from Cyclone Ike. They had nine feet of water go over the top of the peninsula, and the town has never recovered. Pop was born in Abbeville, Louisiana, one of the towns I'll be going through, and he turned out to be a pretty good bloke with a wealth of local knowledge.

There are more bugs now. I was dodging dragonflies all morning, and then the last six miles there was a swarm of bugs getting caught in my "grill." At least they weren't bees, and these little guys were harmless anyway.

High Island is the town I'm staying in tonight, which is thirty-eight feet above sea level built up on a dome of salt. I can see the Gulf of Mexico – fishing boats trawling, more dolphins, birds working, and way out on the horizon – drilling platforms.

The Gulfway Motel is interesting (same lady that answered the phone when I called yesterday). As I'm paying for my room, another traveler finds out the restaurant is closed tonight and the closest one is five miles back. But there is a convenience store next door and that will work for me.

My room door is an aluminum shop front door with the glass painted white. When I open the door, I get the damp wet smell. I'm thinking, "Huge mistake," but I do need a shower. I put on the AC, open the windows, and hit the shower. The shower is great, the towels are clean, and the bed linen is clean. This will work out fine. I've stayed in worse, and it's better than camping in a tent after you have been riding for six hours.

BTW: I've only camped out one night since starting this journey, so I take my hat off to those who have camped out all the way along such an adventure.

Here's today's food log:

Breakfast 1:
one 8 oz white coffee
one banana

Breakfast 2:
one Jack in the Box meat lover's burrito
two 8 oz orange juices
one 8 oz white coffee

Snack:
one PowerBar
one Gatorade
one Bluebell ice cream, covered in chocolate caramel and nuts
two strips of beef jerky

Lunch:
one tin of sardines in tomato sauce
one 24 oz can of Modelo Especial cerveza (beer)
one pack of Mexican chili-lime chips

Dinner:
one chicken potpie
one beefsteak pie
one 24 oz can of Corona Extra

Tonight's my last night in Texas. It's taken 900 miles of riding and more than ten days to get across this enormous state. I've met a lot of great people along the way. I have a better understanding of their history, and leave with a true appreciation and admiration for the Lone Star State of Texas.

Tomorrow I'll be exploring Louisiana, working my way through Cajun country and the swamplands.

Stats for the Day:

Distance travelled – 97 miles/156 kilometers
Average speed – 14.1 mph/22.07 kph
Time – 6 hours 51 minutes
Calories burned – 6,230

The Route:

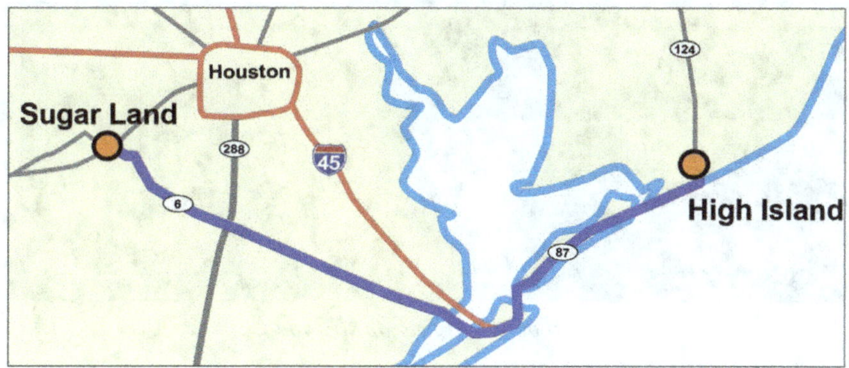

From Sugarland to High Island, Texas.

Pictures of the Day:

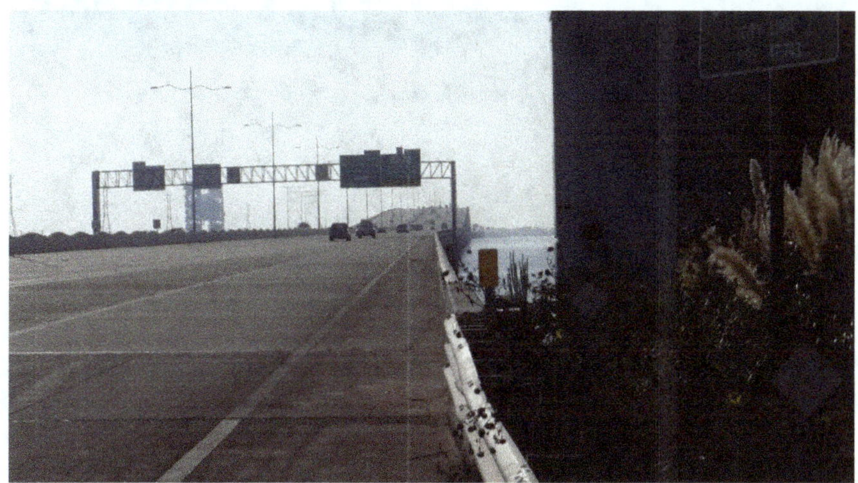

The start of the causeway bridge to Galveston Island.

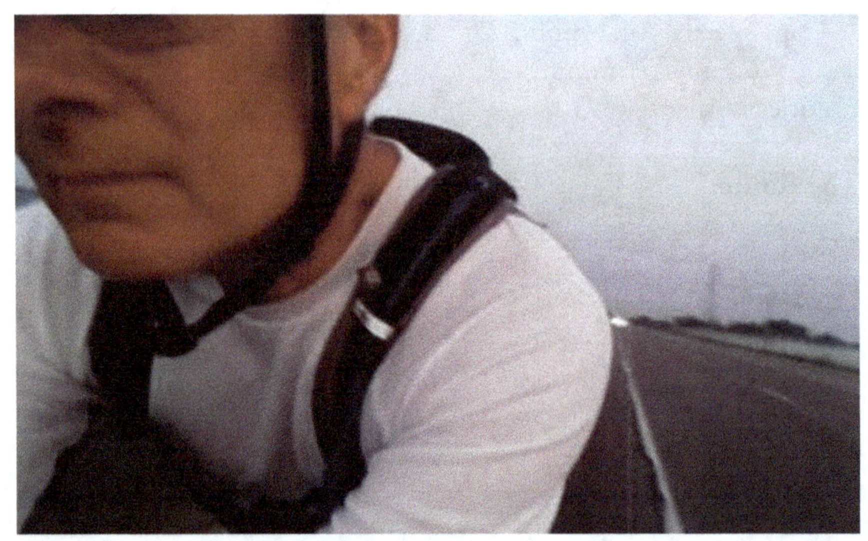

Nice shoulder riding on this road. :)

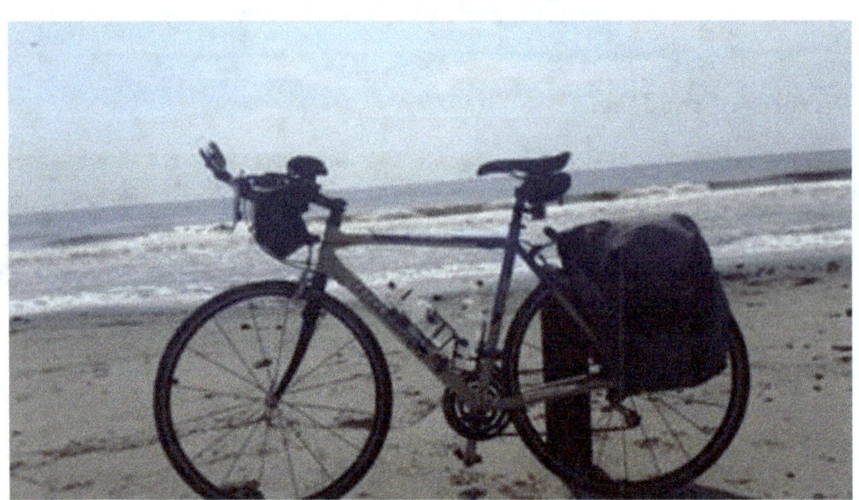

My first beach along the Gulf of Mexico.

Day 4: Tuesday, September 23, 2014

High Island, Texas to Cameron, Louisiana – 98.5 miles/157 kilometers

Silly. Crazy! Why? That's what's running through my head at four this morning. And looking out the window, seeing the hotel flags blowing in the wrong direction, just adds more credibility to my thoughts.

I didn't take a lot of notice when I was checking into the hotel yesterday, but I saw a sign on the counter that had pictures of cockroaches, comparing large and small. This morning there are three "small" cockroaches playing in my bath. No big deal. I turned on the tap and washed them back down the drain. It's only the "big" ones that I can't stand.

I'm soon on Highway 24 and about fifteen miles into the day. I'm riding through Anahuac National Wildlife Refuge, real flat and grassy with nothing around for miles. Good time for a faux coffee (coffee-flavored gel pack). There's no moon and no traffic so I turn off my lights just to see how dark it is. Wow, clear sky and lots of stars!

By sunup I've already had breakfast in Winnie, Texas, where I connect with Interstate 10, which heads northeast to Beaumont, Texas. I'm not taking the Interstate, but instead I'm on Highway 73 heading to Port Arthur. About halfway along, it's time for the first round of sunscreen and another snack. My bike is performing well and everything has settled in for the trip.

Ten miles south of Port Arthur, I cross the T. B. Ellison Parkway Bridge, and I'm now in Louisiana on Highway 82. I'm going through the Sabine National Wildlife Refuge and the roadway is excellent. Hardly any traffic and the drivers are all giving me plenty of room as they pass. That's nice!

There are more wide-open swamps on either side of the road now, but I have my head down focusing on the white line and trying to get an advantage over the headwind. Out of nowhere, the high grass and bamboo completely open up to miles of beach. Small waves, glistening in the sun, roll up the beach. This is the time for a break to take it all in. The road travels along the beach for 20 miles before coming into Holly Beach, a small collection of trailers and homes on poles.

I've been thinking about a Coke for the last ten miles when I see a sign advertising fresh crab and cold drinks. More signs direct me back to an area of mobile homes and a trailer. It's kind of rough looking, but I need a Coke! There's a man and woman talking in their local accent who welcome me. When I ask for a drink, she takes me back to a cool room and says, "In the fridge down the back." I'm about three steps into the cool room and realize the lady is now behind me, holding the door. I instantly think, "Big mistake!" I get a cold Coke from the rack, turn around, and she still has the door open. Sigh of relief . . .

It turns out Meaux's Seafood was ground zero for Hurricane Rita in 2005 and Hurricane Ike in 2008. Sonny is cooking crab and Loretta gets me to sign their guest book. She wouldn't take any money for the Coke, so I left $5 in their guest book.

I push on and catch the ferry into Cameron, Louisiana. The Cameron Motel is right there, but there's another sign that grabs my attention advertising fresh-caught, never-frozen shrimp, just one mile ahead. I think to myself, "*That* will be dinner tonight!"

I check into the hotel and do my routine (shower, wash clothes, recharge light and other electronics). That sign coming into town, "Fresh Shrimp – Never Frozen," is on my mind. I jump back on the bike and head off in search of this feast.

I never found the owner of the sign, but riding along the dock, I see a guy on the back of a trawler peeling shrimp. He sees me and we give each other the nod (I'm too far away to talk to him at this point). A little closer, I ask, "Hey, mate, do you have any fresh shrimp for sale?"

"No, but the captain has plenty at his place we caught last night."

He invites me on board and offers me to try the shrimp he is peeling for his Cajun spaghetti shrimp dinner. "Fresh from the river last night – go on, help yourself." You're kidding me! I'm in heaven right now eating fresh shrimp on a boat in Louisiana!

Beau is sixty-one years old, a born-and-bred Cajun, semi-retired, and goes out shrimping at night. After a tour of the boat, I offer to pay for the shrimp. He tells me, "I'll take $1.65 if you have it. That will buy me a beer."

I said, "I would gladly give you that, but I only have a twenty." He points to the gas station across the road that sells beer. I follow him over on the bike, I break the twenty and try to buy him a six-pack, but all he wanted was two 24 oz cans of Miller High Life.

What a great day after all. Seriously, you can't make this stuff up!

Stats for the Day:

Distance travelled – 98.55 miles/157 kilometers
Average speed – 12.4 mph/20 kph
Time – 7 hours 39 minutes
Calories burned – 5,683

The Route:

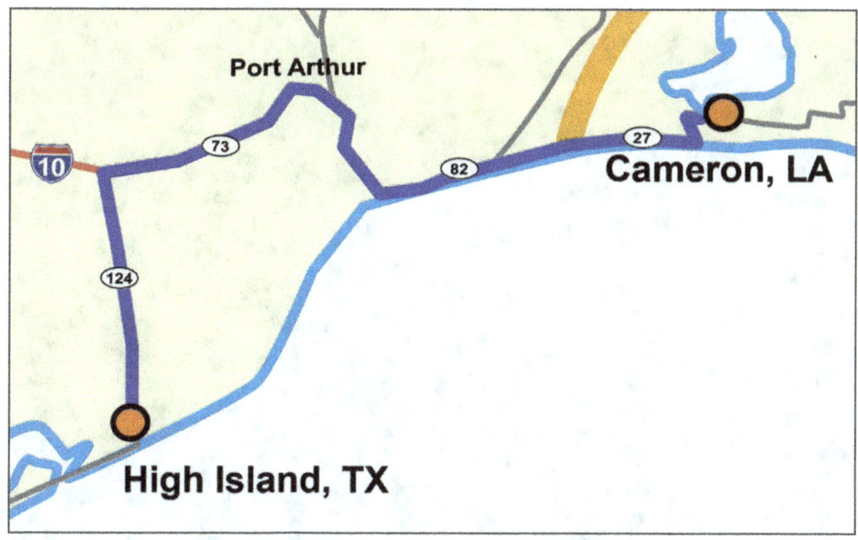

From High Island, Texas, to Cameron, Louisiana.

Pictures of the Day:

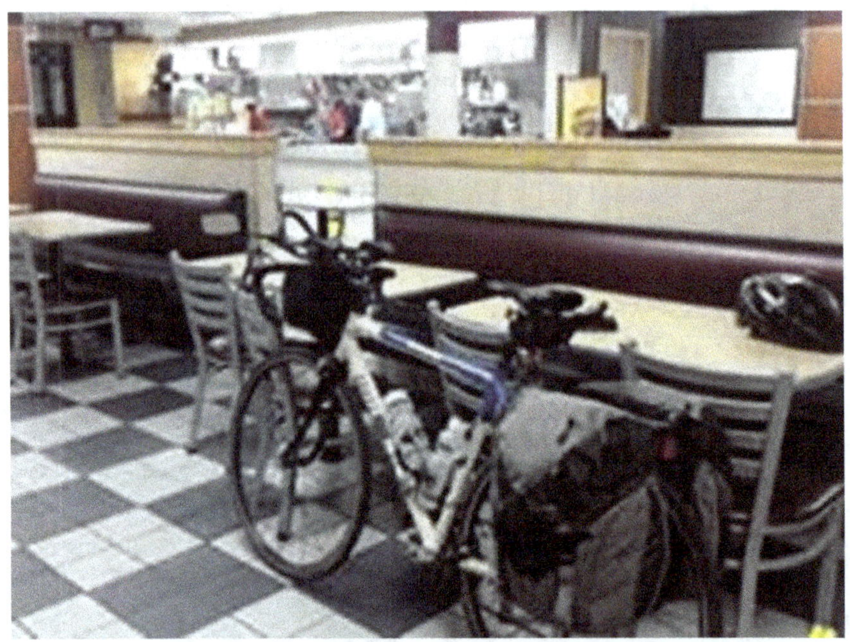

"A number 7, thanks!" – breakfast at McDonald's.

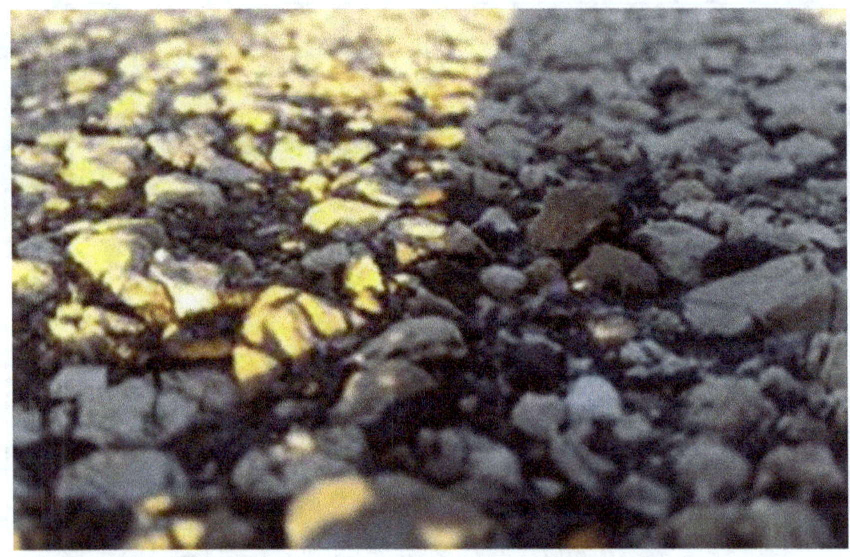

Close-up shot of the chip seal road surface – not good for the knees.

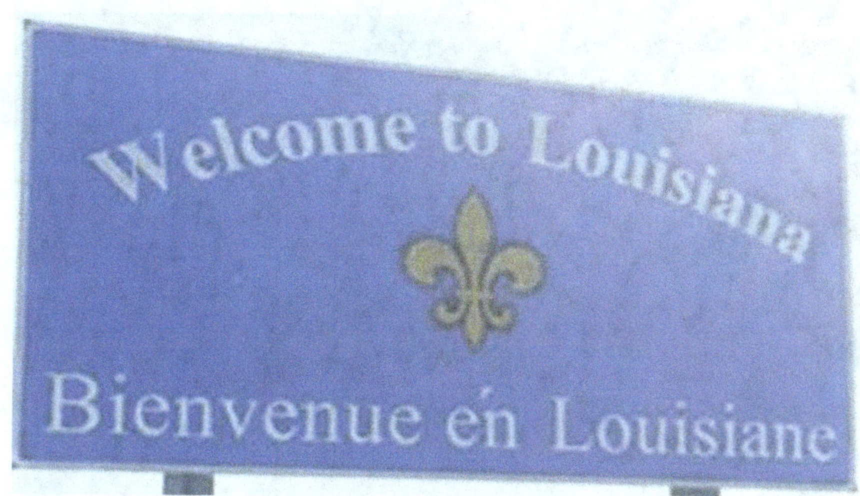

Finally out of Texas.

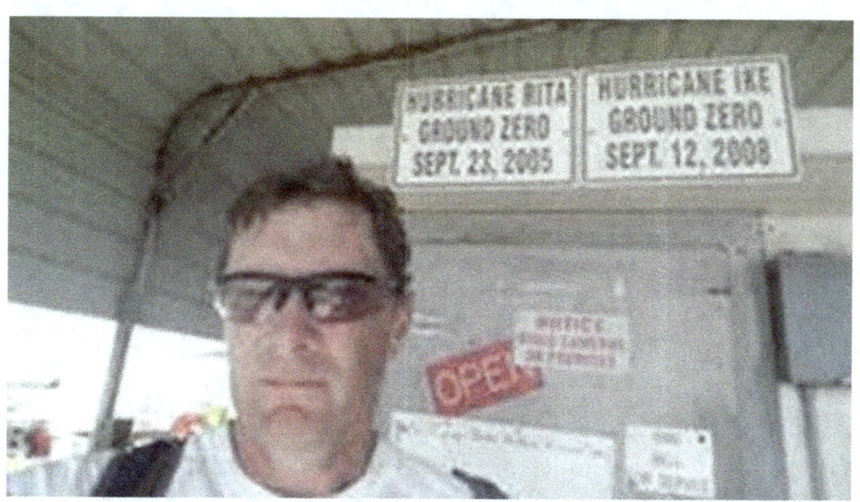

Holly Beach – Meaux's Seafoods. Cooler door in the background.

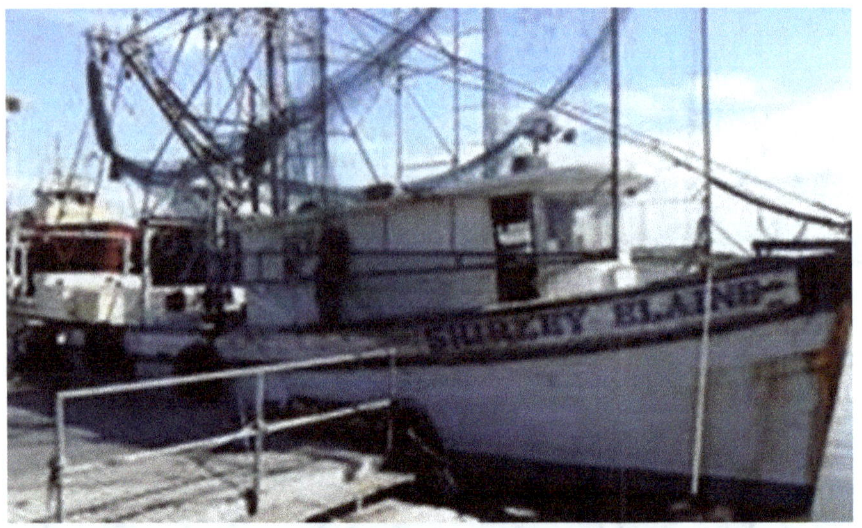

The Shirley Elaine shrimp boat.

Day 5: Wednesday, September 24, 2014

Cameron to Abbeville, Louisiana – 100.5 miles/162 kilometers

Wow! This was another big day, just over 100 miles. Let's just add this up: almost 500 miles over 5 days, burning over 30,000 calories and 36 hours in the saddle. My body is like a machine at the moment. I feel electric and charged with unstoppable energy! Everything is working like it should except for a couple of sore areas, as you would imagine. I just hope I can keep up the pace for two more days and the 156 miles to New Orleans. We will see.

Sipping my gel pack coffee this morning while cruising in the dark, I got to thinking about the shrimp boat last night and *Forrest Gump*. That boat could have been the *Jenny* from the movie, with Captain Dan struggling to get around on the deck in his wheelchair after his legs got blown off in the war. Next, I'm thinking about Forrest Gump and how he started running with no real reason, to the point where he had a bunch of followers. Maybe they were similar to all you couch cruisers and armchair riders. By the way, couch cruising is one of the other things that I'm really good at and practice quite a bit! The point is, maybe those people that were following him helped motivate him to continue to run. It's like your emails of encouragement, and just the fact that I know you are reading this stuff is motivating me! Run, Forrest, run!

I'm in the middle of Rockefeller State Wildlife Refuge and it's another perfect sunrise. It's time to welcome the day, apply sunscreen, and enjoy breakfast by the side of the road. There aren't many stores along the road, so I have my own provisions – a tin of sardines and a cold bottle of Gatorade. Okay, it doesn't sound like these two things should go together, but it tasted great and filled the need. Next time, I need to have toast with the sardines.

This part of the country is beautiful with water everywhere, everything green, and endless seafood. The roads are well maintained and in great condition, as they are part of the hurricane evacuation route. If you have not ventured down this way, it's really worth a trip. Take your time and enjoy Cameron's fishing town and the wildlife parks in the area. Go take a ride on an airboat through the swamp. That's what I'm doing on my next visit and which will be in or on *something with a motor*!

I heard a few pops this morning. Tires look good. Hmm . . . My lower back is fine, my knees all good. It turns out to be people hunting in the swamp. I pull into Pecan Island's only store for my second breakfast. I was talking to the girl behind the counter about the popping sounds. She told me that they are filming *Swamp People* this week and the gunshots probably came from that. Apparently, the show's headers – Liz, Jason, Jay-Paul, and the guy wearing the overalls – all live around here and come in the store all the time. They are selling "Choot Em" shirts signed by Liz and the rest of the cast. How about that! Just a small town of hunting camps surrounded by swamp, and now part of a national TV reality show.

Tonight I have a business dinner with one of my dealers. John runs the professional services division in the Big South Area. I've known him for years, a great guy and true Cajun. John is keen to see my bike, so I bring it into the foyer of the hotel. He holds the bike with one hand on the seat and the other on the handlebars. He looks at me and says, "I can feel the energy!" It must be some Cajun witchcraft he was feeling, but I'm now a believer.

One of the best things about this adventure is the ability to mix it with business. Prior to leaving, I'd pack my carry-on roller bag, just like any business trip, with my suits, shirts, ties, etc. Then I'd package the roller bag in a cardboard box and have it delivered to my last hotel. This way, when I arrived at the last hotel, I would have all my business attire to meet customers in that area.

From San Diego and now in Louisiana, I have enjoyed the company of many business associates and new friends along the way. Thanks for the hospitality in your hometowns – Dave, Ron, Andreas, Bob, Dan, and John.

To Mark, from Precision Bikes in Lafayette, thanks for the input on Highway 82. It's a great road for bicycling!

Morgan City tomorrow . . .

Stats for the Day:

Distance travelled – 100.5 miles/162 kilometers
Average speed – 14 mph/23 kph
Time – 7 hours
Calories burned – 6,321

The Route:

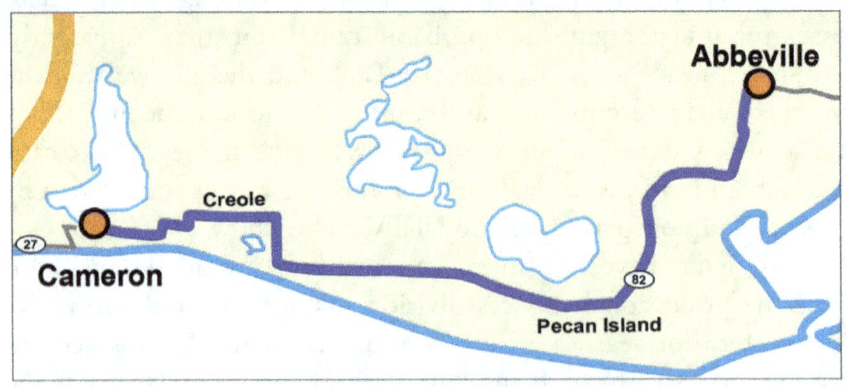

From Cameron to Abbeville, Louisiana.

Pictures of the Day:

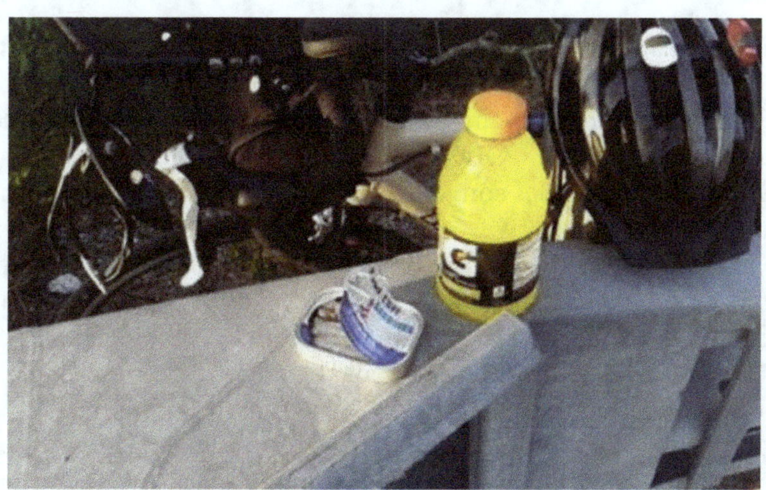

Breakfast – sardines and Gatorade.

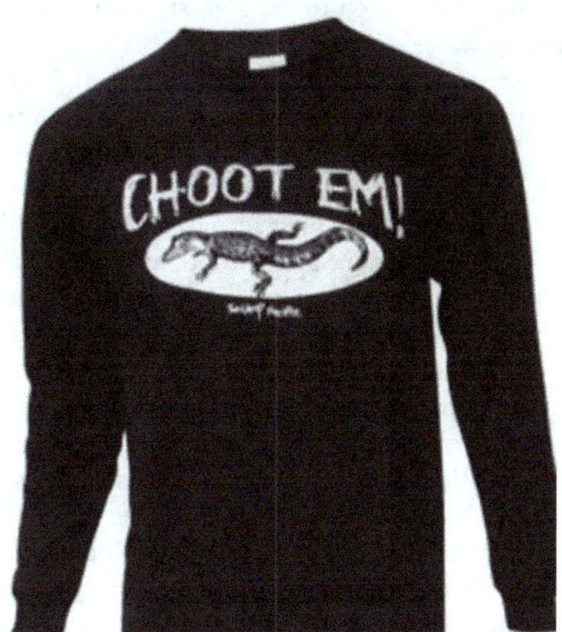

Gear from the show Swamp People.

Day 6: Thursday, September 25, 2014

Abbeville to Morgan City, Louisiana – 70.4 miles/113 kilometers

There are not as many miles today, as there are no in-between hotel stops before New Orleans that don't take me out of my way. I ended up with 70 miles completed today and now I'm only 90 miles from finishing tomorrow.

I left the hotel just before 6:00 a.m. with a reasonable breakfast. About 15 miles along Highway 14, I'm cycling through the town of Delcambre, the heartland of Cajun Acadiana. The biggest thing in this town is their drawbridge, one of the largest I've seen so far. I'm also sweating out the Louisiana Abita's I enjoyed last night.

Andrew Zimmern (a.k.a. Bizarre Foods) is 100 percent right. Bugs do taste earthy. Just around sunrise there they are, always waiting for me to take a big breath. I've been pretty lucky, only getting one or two in the mouth or nose, but today . . . As I suck that morning air in . . . Yep, it's enough to get a good sample, quickly followed by a mouthful of water to rinse out.

I'm just south of New Iberia following Highway 90, which cuts through the middle of sugarcane plantations. You can see on a map these plantations are surrounded by swamps and waterways. Sometimes highways will have a frontage road that runs parallel to the highway (I call them "bicycle retreats") away from the eighteen-wheelers. This one is nice and smooth and the occasional tractor passes to keep me entertained. A stick of sugarcane falls from one of the tractors, so I stop, pick it up, and cut a piece off to chew on. If you haven't tried this, don't expect to get a mouth full of sugar. It's like chewing on bamboo, but does have a sweet taste.

Mate, I have to tell you, going through these small rural towns, I'm starting to feel like a bitch on heat! They must be able to *smell* me coming along the road. I had at least half a dozen good sprints against dogs today. I saw a kennel with a doorway that looked big enough for a bear! Luckily, I didn't have to go to maneuver no. 3 (pepper spray) or need to get off my bike. I think I'm getting used to them now. Maybe I'd make a good mail deliverer (or postman in Australia).

I worked out today that everything on my bike is round. I can't think of anything that is square. No, even that! It's round, too! Yep, everything's round!

Franklin is a small town just before Morgan City. It's just like you would expect to see down here: southern style mansions, great gardens and streets lined with Spanish moss trees hanging over the road. Very quaint, but it's time for more food!

I see them as I pull up and rest my bike against the window. They are watching me with curiosity and talking amongst themselves. I don't make any eye contact. I keep to myself. I order a number 7 meal, which in this town is now a number 11 meal. A family ordering their breakfast tells me they saw me on Highway 90 this morning and ask, "Where are you going? Where did you come from? What is the cause?" They're blown away with my story and I know *they* are listening. I sit down to eat and position myself where I can see my bike and also see *them*. They are talking about medical procedures and prescription drugs. I know one of them is going to start up at any minute. Sure enough . . . "Where are you going, where ya from, and why?" It's the old guy's morning coffee club at McDonald's. Half a dozen of them have rapid-fire questions for me. One guy has an accent that is so thick his mate has to repeat stuff for him.

Things start to settle down when I tell them they drive better than those Texans. Another one of the morning coffee club pipes up, "So where are you from?

"I rode from Abbeville." They are impressed. Then I say, "From San Antonio last Saturday . . . but started in San Diego . . . I live in Phoenix . . . and I'm from Australia."

Now we are all confused. Where am I from and why am I doing this? This is more food for thought while riding. By the way, the one guy with the real thick accent recently had a stroke that affected his speech and that's why his mate was translating for him.

Around 11:45 a.m., I cross the old bridge over the Atchafalaya River. In the picture below, you can see the flood walls and gates that circle the city. I'm cycling through the back streets of the city in a pretty run-down area, then, oh no, another sign for fresh seafood and this time boiled crab! The place is falling apart, been there for years, and so has Roy behind the counter. He sells rabbit meat, crab, alligator steaks, and just about any other thing that moves. See pictures below.

"Do you have any crabs, mate?"

"Huh? Not till one thirty. They're out back cooking right now."

Damn. That's another hour and a half and the hotel is five miles ahead. I cannot add ten more miles to this trip, so Roy's crab will have to wait for next time. What a coincidence. It turns out that Roy used to drive the ferryboat from Galveston to Bolivar point twenty years ago. He tells me about how it was down there along the peninsula before the big hurricanes. He gave me a nice tour of his store that has a collection of oddball items, pictures, and news clippings gathered over the years. Did you know that there is a fish that has a head like an alligator that's called an alligator-gar? Interesting. Roy has the skulls of both species and explains the differences. He's really quite the character.

One more day with 90 miles and I will hopefully take my prize – arriving in the French Quarter on famous Bourbon Street, New Orleans. However, the icing on the cake is that I will be meeting up with Sara for the weekend and sharing all the other stories and pictures from this awesome trip.

Stats for the Day:

Distance travelled – 70 miles/113 kilometers
Average speed – 13 mph/21 kph
Time – 5 hours 15 minutes
Calories burned – 4,231

The Route:

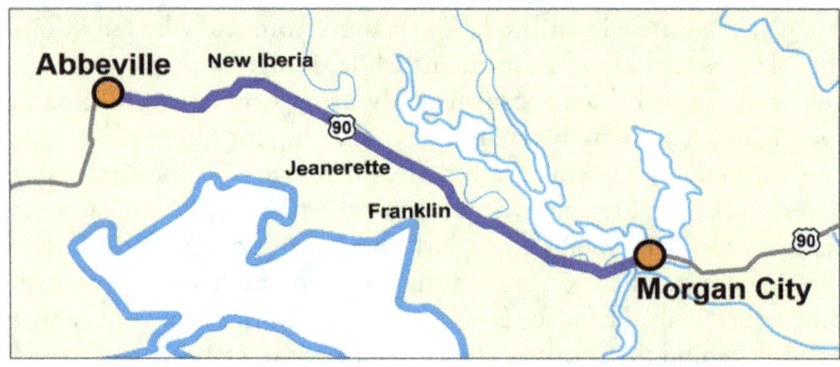

From Abbeville to Morgan City, Louisiana.

Pictures of the Day:

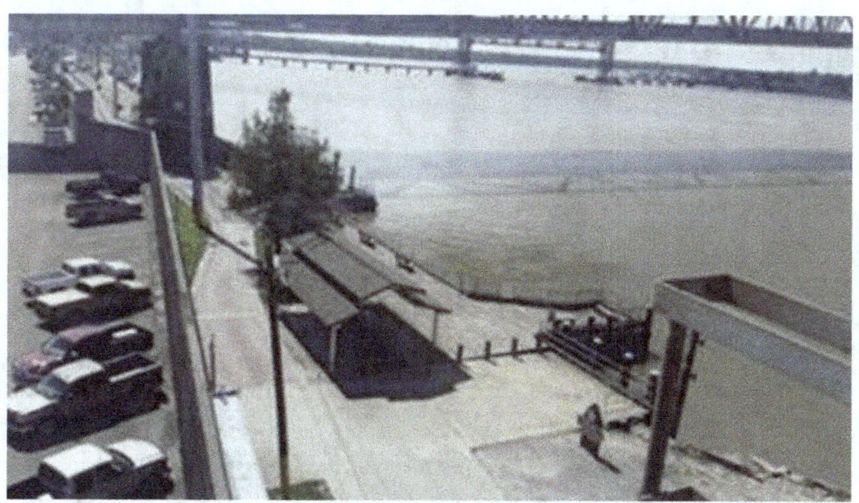

Flood walls and gate along the Atchafalaya River.

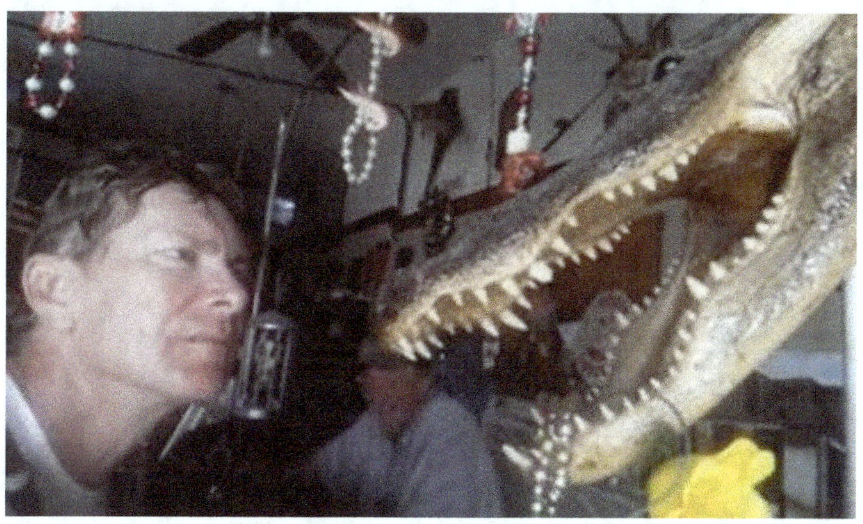

That's definitely a gator!

Day 7: Friday, September, 26, 2014

**Morgan City to New Orleans, Louisiana – 92 miles/148 kilometers
THE BIG EASY**

Last night's dinner was a choice between the Chef's Surprise that comes with two beers for $15 or some other known pasta dish for $16 without two beers. Seems like an easy decision, right? It turns out the Chef's Surprise was fettuccine and shrimp in cream sauce and two local beers of my choice. Right up my alley and a great meal, which I reflected on the survey that came with it.

During dinner, while studying the maps, I'm really torn whether to ride the back road (rough with little to no shoulder and more crazy dogs) or take Highway 90 (a better road with a good shoulder but duking it out with the eighteen-wheelers). To help in the decision process, I called the local police station. The officer informed me there was no law against cycling on Highway 90, but the back road would probably be safer. Big decision, right?

It's 5:30 a.m., dark, and I'm on Highway 90 making a beeline into New Orleans, excited to see the Mississippi River. Although the road has a great shoulder, I'm dodging lots of roadside debris and something new – bump strips. These are just like the reflectors on the shoulder of the roadway except these are put on a forty-five-degree angle across the shoulder of the approaches to each bridge. In this part of the world, there are many, many bridges. I guess the idea is to alert motorists that they are coming up to a bridge and it may be icy in the winter weather. Well, on a bike in Autumn, they become a game of lining up your bike tires to squeeze between them at 16–18 miles an hour. It takes full concentration to navigate these along with the rocks, nails, and screws. Now and then you will clip one and feel the impact through the bike.

Nothing could stop me today. Even a flat tire before daylight wasn't a problem. *Pop* (or more like a *ping*) . . . I stop and check the front tire. All good here. I start pedaling and realize it's the rear tire, of course. A huge piece of metal had gone right through my new Continental Gatorskin tire. It was the quickest rear tire change I've ever done. I take the luggage off and the back wheel off and find the hole. It's too dark for patching the tube and the hole was too big anyway. By this time I've attracted the attention of the only locals awake this time of the morning and they are hungry. News spreads fast and soon I'm in a cloud of mosquitoes. A great incentive to get moving and quickly!

As daylight appears, I'm in Schriever, Louisiana, about 26 miles along from Morgan City. I stop at the first gas station to clean the chain grease off my hands. It's perfect timing for a coffee, cheese Danish, and a banana. There's a guy selling fruit. I wander over for a chat. He thinks I'm from Austria and starts telling me about his German heritage. "No worries, mate, I'll take a bag of that alligator jerky," I say and I'm away again. Not bad jerky, really tastes good.

I pass through Boutte, Louisiana, on the outskirts of the city and am now only 30 miles from New Orleans. This takes me right to the Mississippi and I'm cycling along a path that runs along the top of the river's levy banks. I have a clear view of the city and the river. There is lots of commercial boat traffic, but in the middle of this, I see a nice old paddle steamer making its way along the river. Beautiful.

It's a little breezy and soon I'm crossing my last bridge. It's a monumental bridge called the Huey P. Long (yes, that is the name of the bridge), and it takes me into New Orleans. I have about nine miles of cycling through the city to get to the French Quarter. Trams go by and the smell of restaurants at lunchtime fills the air. I pass by Louisiana State University and blend in with all the other bicyclists on the road.

Finally, I'm on the corner of Conti and Bourbon Streets and have finished a very memorable ride. I need some beads, a beer or two, and a bath!

Stats for the Day:

Distance travelled – 92 miles/148 kilometers
Average speed – 14 mph/22.7 kph
Time – 6 hours 20 minutes
Calories burned – 5,792

The Route:

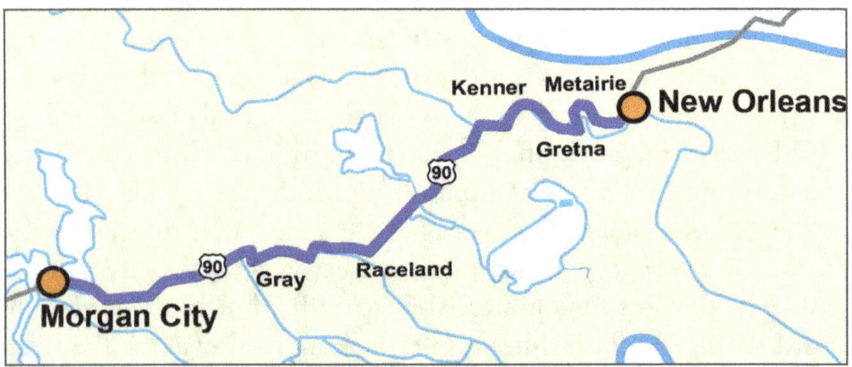

From Morgan City to New Orleans, Louisiana.

Pictures of the Day:

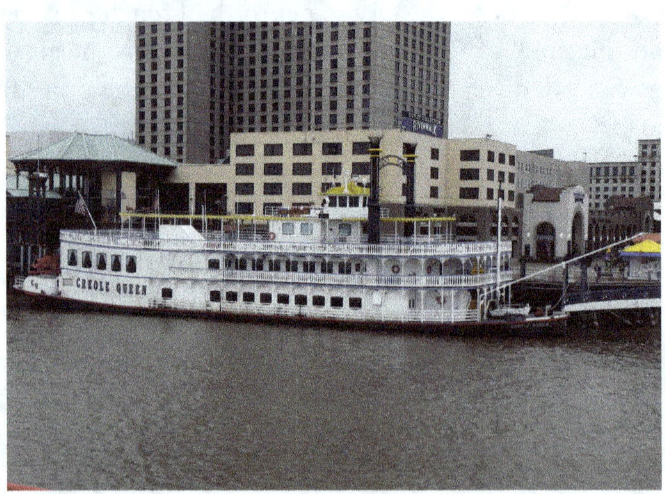

Famous Mississippi Paddle Steamer Natchez

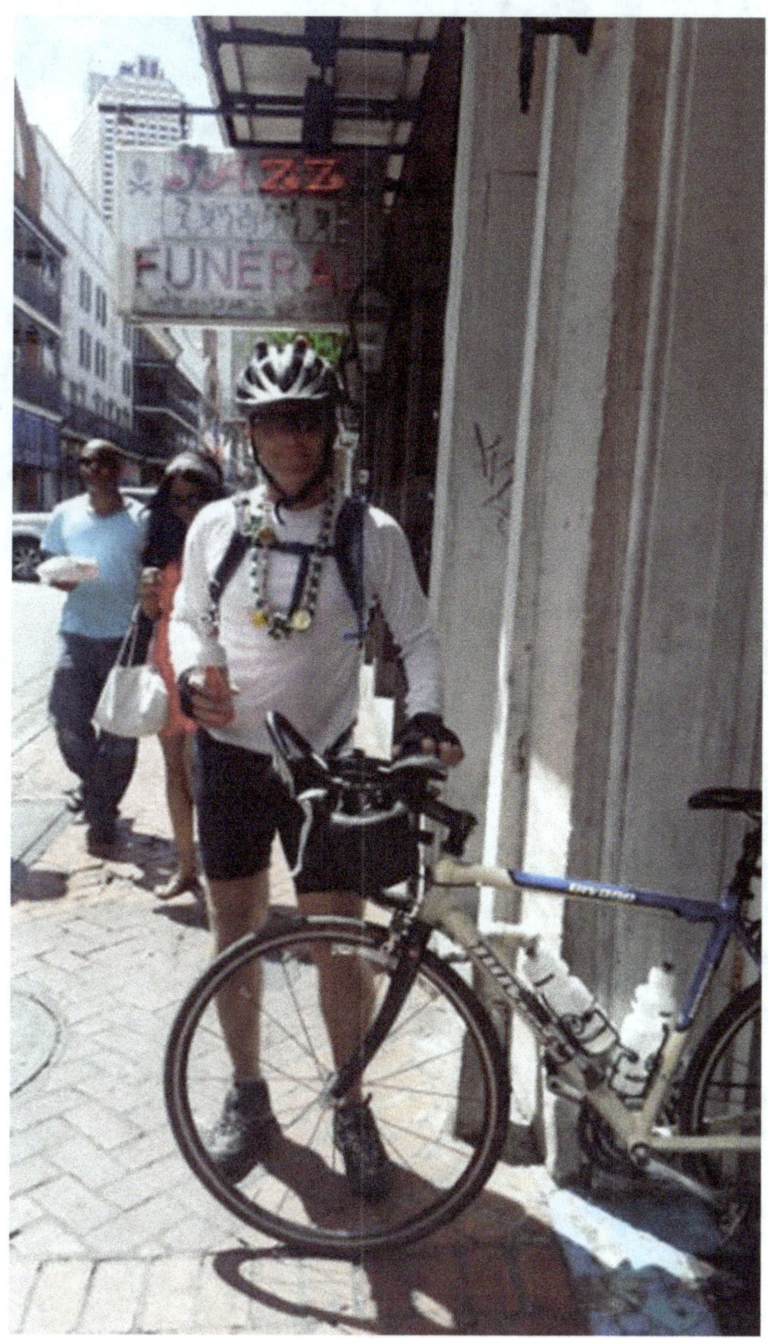

On the corner of Bourbon and Conti Streets,
New Orleans French Quarter.

Some feedback on the car spotted on Day 1:

John – Around a 1974 Plymouth Satellite Roadrunner
Susan – Between 1978–1980 Plymouth Roadrunner.
Bill – 1964 Chevelle
Clay – '73 Roadrunner
Tom – Dodge Charger
Peter – 1973 Dodge Challenger
David – Plymouth Roadrunner
Ron – '60s vintage Dodge Charger
Eddie – '72 Challenger
Rich – 1969 Plymouth

The correct answer:

1973 Plymouth Road Runner

1973 Plymouth Roadrunner

See original listing

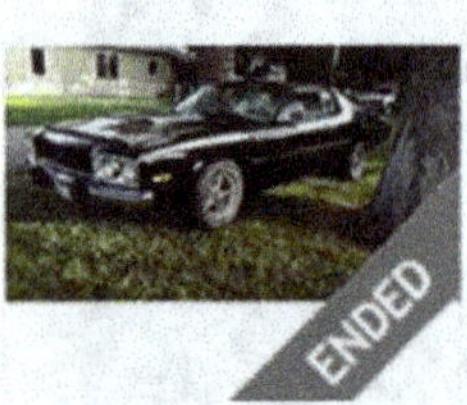

Item condition:	**Used**
Ended:	Aug 11, 2014 8/11, 2:35PM
Starting bid:	**US $18,500.00** [0 bids]
Shipping:	Will ship to United States. Read item options.
Item location:	Shiner, Texas, United States

CHAPTER 6

New Orleans, Louisiana to St. Augustine, Florida
November 1–7, 2015

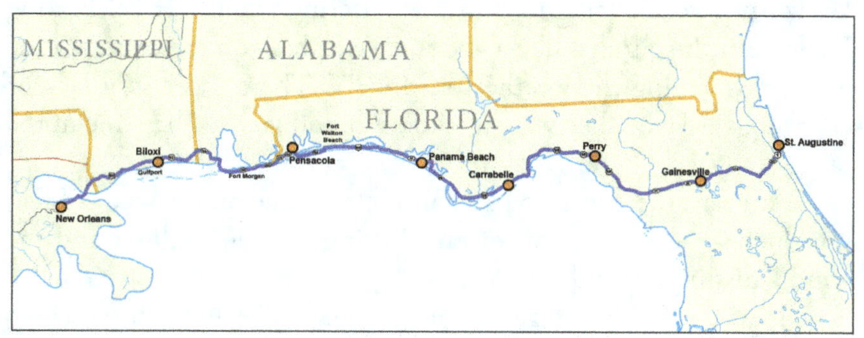

Total distance – 681 miles/1,096 kilometers
Number of days – 7 days
Average speed – 14.8 mph/ 23.8 kph
Total saddle time – 46 hours, 35 minutes

Day 1: Sunday, November 1, 2015

New Orleans, Louisiana to Biloxi, Mississippi – 102 miles/164 kilometers

Really glad that day is *done*!

I was out of the hotel at daybreak, 7:00 a.m. The girl at the front desk took a picture and commented on how wet it was going to be today. She wasn't kidding. It was windy and rained all day except for the last 15 miles where it was windy and just sprinkling. I was probably due for a wet day; it's only the second wet day I've had since starting the adventure. It's been twenty-seven days of sun versus two wet days.

It was pretty much eight hours in the rain with the wind from the northeast, of course. The upside was that most people stayed home, maybe because of a football game, LSU (Louisiana State University) versus (?), and possibly suffering from over celebrating Halloween. It sounded like a good place to be – on the couch in the warmth watching the weather on the TV. There was also a lack of crazy dogs. Maybe they were just too wet and lazy to chase me in the rain.

Anyway, there was no jazz band to send me on my way as I had imagined – just the sound of rain hitting my bike helmet and the wind whistling around my ears.

It was difficult navigating out of the city. A wet phone screen is like having ten fingers doing ten different things and not much help when everything is wet. My course was taking me along the top of the levee banks that hold back Lake Pontchartrain. This was too windy, so I moved down and cycled through the neighborhoods, twisting and turning while keeping the wind on my left front side as a guide for directions.

These streets are a patchwork of concrete and potholes covered with varying depths of water and are really slippery. I hit a pothole really hard and thought, "Wow! I can't believe I didn't get a flat tire." Within one second I feel it – a flat and it's on the back. Really, this is going to be a *long* day. On a positive note, it's easier to change out a tube and refit a tire when everything is wet and greasy.

Eventually, I find Highway 90 and am now clear of the city. It's just me and the weather. Passing through the bayous there are a bunch of fishing camps with houses built up high on poles, like back on the Texas Gulf coast, due to all the hurricanes.

I was planning on staying in Gulf Port, but got a few extra miles in and finished the day in Biloxi, Mississippi. I'm *so* glad to be out of my wet gear!

Stats for the Day:

Distance travelled – 102 miles/164.15 kilometers
Average speed – 13 mph/20.9 kph
Time – 7 hours 51 minutes
Calories burned – 6,300

The Route:

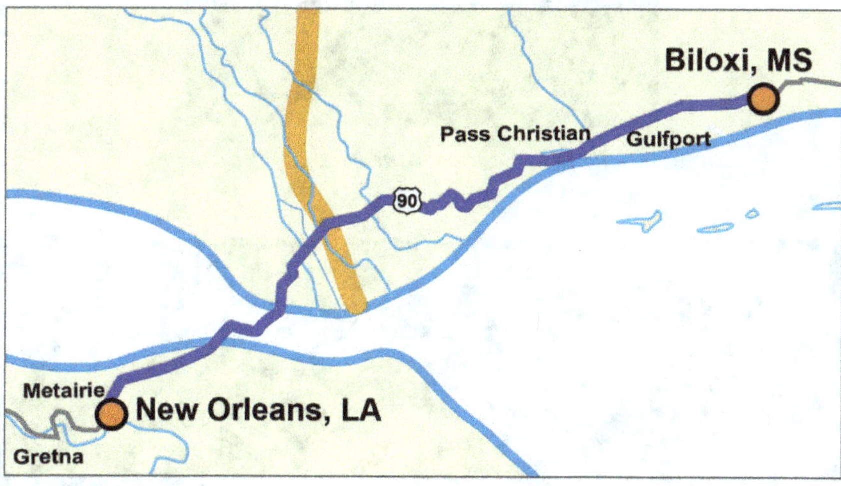

From New Orleans, Louisiana, to Biloxi, Mississippi.

Pictures of the Day:

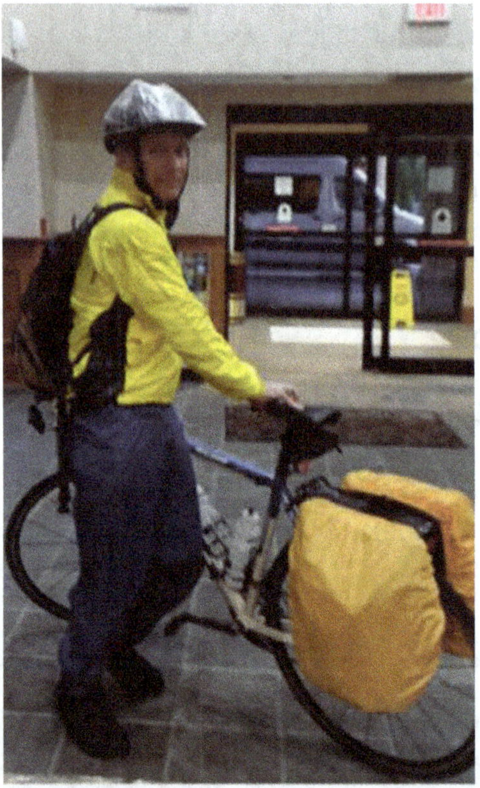

Finally found a use for the hotel shower cap.

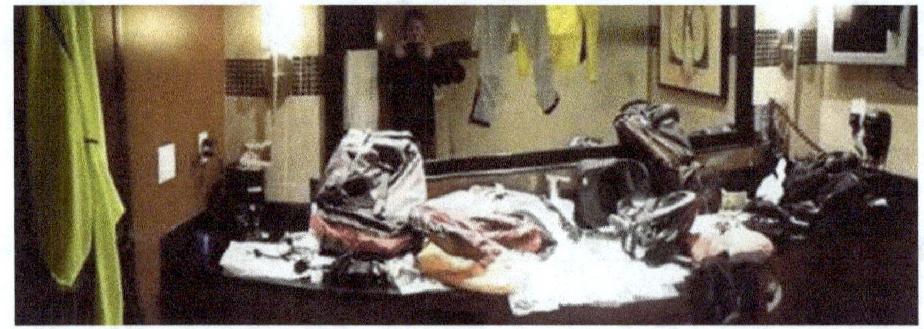

Notice the hair dryer to the right drying my shoes . . . and everything else.

Day 2: Monday, November 2, 2015

Biloxi, Mississippi to Pensacola, Florida – 124 miles/200 kilometers

I'm always amazed how one day can be so incredibly difficult and the next day just phenomenal.

Tonight I'm in Pensacola, Florida, after blowing through Mississippi and Alabama. The weather today was excellent with sunshine all day and a nice wind from the southwest. It feels like having a hand on the back of my saddle firmly pushing me along versus a headwind, which is like a hand on the brake.

Leaving Biloxi this morning, looking out to the Gulf of Mexico, I thought I saw *"Pretty girls dancin' in the sea. They all look like sisters in the ocean."* Who knew that Jimmy Buffett was born is Pascagoula, Mississippi? It's the land of bayous, beaches, bars, boiled crab, burgers with cheese, boats, and beers – pretty much the topics of his music. You can see that influence everywhere you look. The sign entering the state of Mississippi says, *"The Birthplace of American Music."*

I was so tempted to stop in Bayou La Batre, Alabama, this morning and get some of that fresh shrimp I've been longing for, but it was too early and I had just polished off a big breakfast at Macca's about an hour earlier. This little town is known as the *Seafood Capital of Alabama*, and smells like it too. One sign said, *"If it swims, we have it!"*

Rather than go north into Mobile, Alabama, I went south to Dauphin Island, then caught the ferry across Mobile Bay to Fort Morgan. About a mile from the dock, I see a loaded up cyclist making steady progress on the footpath. I give him a wave and continued on knowing that we'd catch-up on the ferry. Jon has ridden through all but two states in the continental US over the last two years. What a champion! He is on his way to Gainesville, Florida, to meet up with a lady friend.

We rode together for 10 miles or so and swapped a few yarns (stories). He had the same two dogs chase him that went after me earlier in the day just before Port Alabama. It's just part of it. You are going to mess with a few dogs here and there. As the traffic picked up, our conversation becomes limited as I was either behind Jon or in front of him to let the cars pass by. We bid each other a safe journey and parted ways.

I was planning on staying in Gulf Shores, Alabama, tonight, but the wind was so good, I took advantage of the situation and completed another 25 miles. I arrived in Pensacola in the Eastern Time zone at 5:15 p.m. Tomorrow, I pray for more of that helping hand from the southwest!

Stats for the Day:

Distance travelled – 124 miles/200 kilometers
Average speed – 16.1 mph/25.9kph
Time – 7 hours 40 minutes
Calories burned – 8,392

The Route:

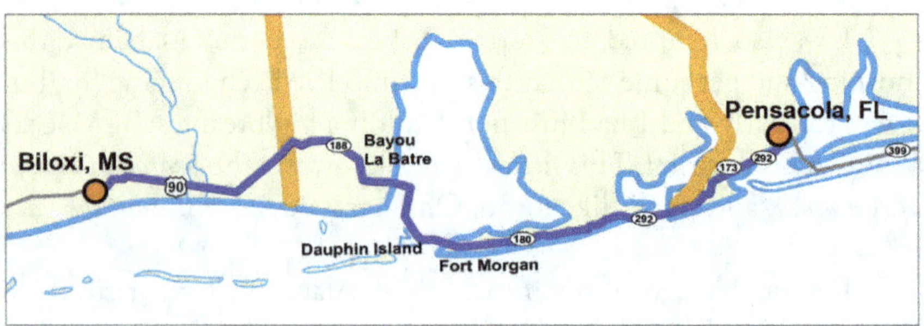

From Biloxi, Mississippi, to Pensacola, Florida.

Pictures of the Day:

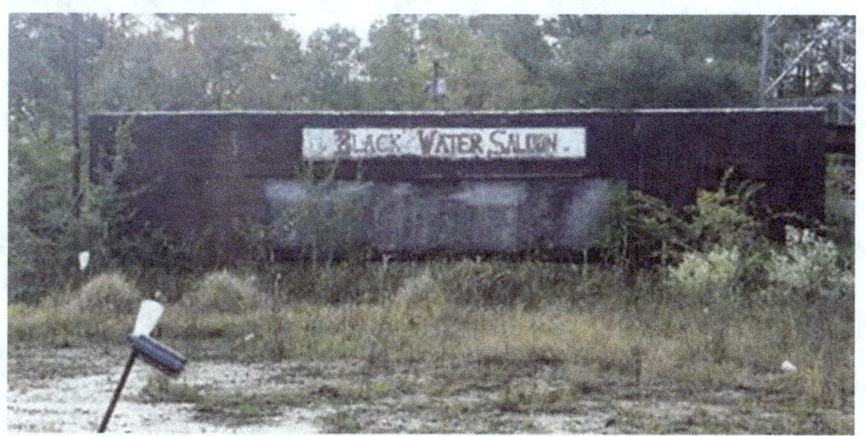

The Pub with No Beer – on the Mississippi-Alabama border.

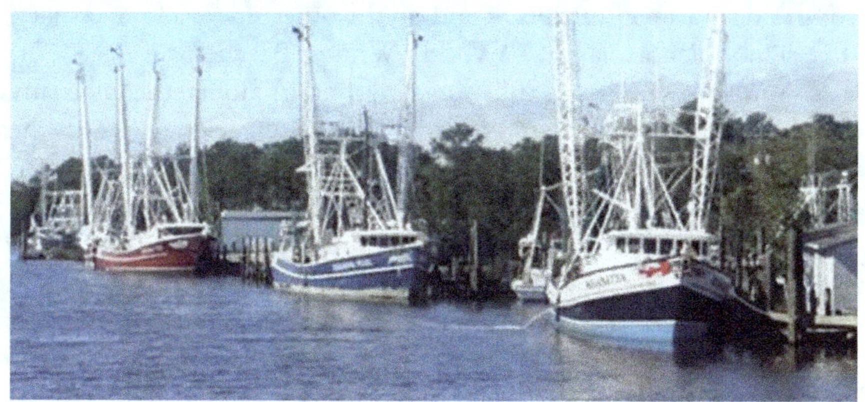

The picturesque town of Bayou La Batre, Alabama.

Day 3: Tuesday, November 3, 2015

Pensacola to Panama Beach, Florida – 101 miles/163 kilometers

Another fine sunny day on the Gulf Coast!

I was on the road at 6:30 a.m. and heavily involved in the morning commute through Pensacola. We all have somewhere to go and some of us at different speeds. I just rode the white line and hugged the gutter, which eventually took me over the Pensacola Bay Bridge. The next bridge was almost void of traffic, providing time to look around and see dolphins swimming in the bay.

Just a few more miles and I'm back on the beach again, working my way through Gulf Island Seashore National Park. The next twenty miles are isolated with maybe one or three cars passing by. The road is partially covered in white sand. Beyond the sand on the south side is a small surf break and on the other side is a long estuary. The sign in Pensacola says, "World's Whitest Beaches."

Sunday's rain and sandy roadways aren't doing the bike any favors. Tom, my mechanic buddy, completely changed out the running gear before this ride and the bike feels like it's brand-new. However, yesterday I noticed a noise when pulling on the back brake, not constant, just each time the wheel turned. That pothole in NOLA (New Orleans, LA) did a number on the back rim; it looked like someone took a hammer and dented it in. It should be fine, but I was really lucky it wasn't worse. If the rim had broken, I would probably be spending the day looking for replacement, but at least I would have been out of the wind and rain. Anyway, I found a car wash and managed to get the bloke running it to pressure wash the running gear and chain. Then I applied a little lube and everything looked brand-new again.

As the morning progressed, I cycled through Fort Walton and on to Okaloosa Island, which is the last primitive area before Destin. From here on in, it's beach houses, condos, and high-rise apartments. It almost looks like you're in Laguna Beach or Santa Monica, California, or the Gold Coast in Australia. They actually have road signs with "Laguna Beach" and "Santa Monica" minus the

California. One place worth a visit, or at least a virtual visit, is Aly's Beach. Check this place out! I thought I was in Anguilla down in the Caribbean known for its beautiful beaches.

Hang on, I'll be right back. I have to go and watch the sunset from my hotel room balcony! Absolutely spectacular as it touches the horizon, spreading its last light for the day across the water. See the picture below.

I arrived in Panama City Beach about 2:00 p.m. The hotel for tonight is holding the Florida Ironman event that starts this weekend, which I thought was very serendipitous, even though I will miss it. I did see a number of professional cyclists on the road about 12 miles from the hotel. These guys were working hard. Completely decked out in all the gear, usually wearing white rimmed sunglasses, and looking very fast, even when stopped at a traffic light. I'm not sure how much more speed you get if you shave your legs, but I really don't care!

One of the bonuses of staying in these low budget hotels is that they haven't changed out the showerheads to the low flows that the midrange hotels use. Nothing's better than a strong hot shower. You think they would advertise this feature, like they do with free Wi-Fi or hotel shuttle, or at least give it an extra star on the ratings.

I'm about 25 miles ahead of schedule and almost halfway through this last section of my ride. Tomorrow I'll move a little slower and hope to finish in Carrabelle, Florida. It looks like another fishing town and more great seafood. Bring it on!

Stats for the Day:

Distance travelled – 100.14 miles/162 kilometers
Average speed – 15.8 mph/ 24.42 kph
Time – 6 hours 20 minutes
Calories burned – 6,759

The Route:

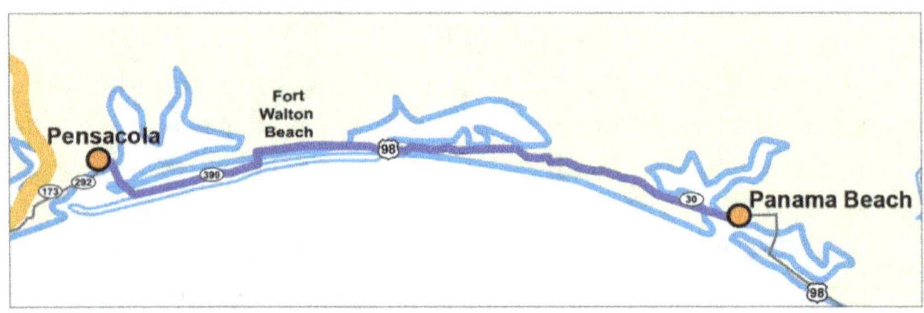

From Pensacola to Panama Beach, Florida.

Pictures of the Day:

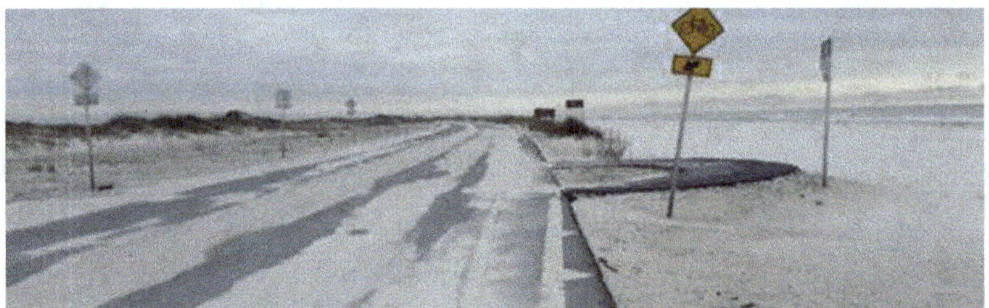

Gulf Island Seashore National Park – just beautiful.

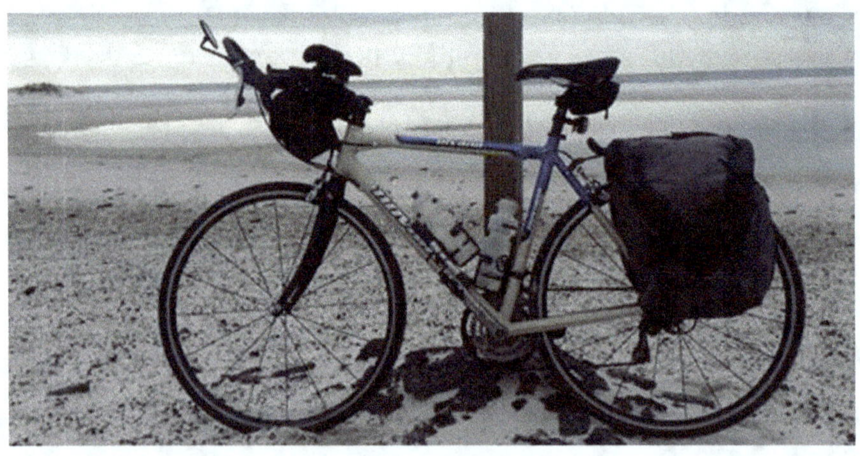

My trusty ride.

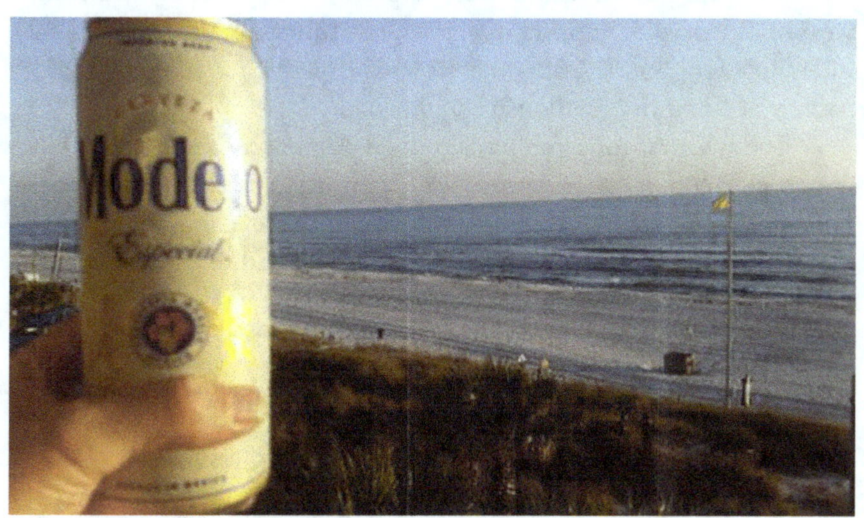

Yes, that is a 24 oz (710 ml) beer in my hand.

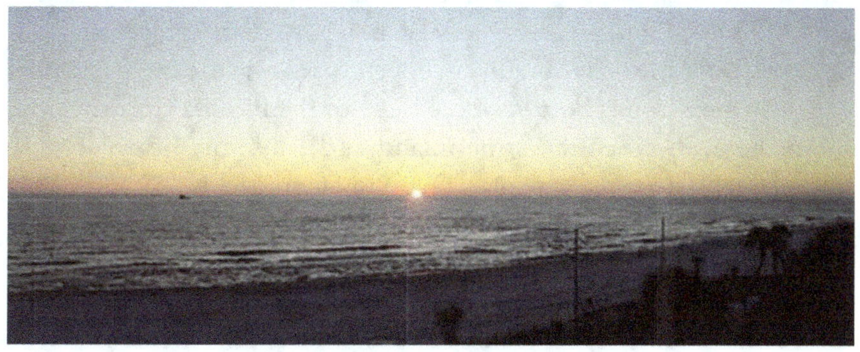

Sunset, just before the green flash.

Day 4: Wednesday, November 4, 2015

Panama Beach to Carrabelle, Florida – 94 miles/151 kilometers

Tonight I'm in Carrabelle, approximately sixty miles southwest of Tallahassee, Florida. Over the last four days, I've covered 421 miles, leaving about 260 miles to my finish line, the edge of the Atlantic Ocean in St. Augustine, Florida.

Today's ride took me past Tyndell Air Force Base, which takes up about half of the 25-mile long peninsula that sits just below Panama City (see map below). The scenery has changed now, and either side of the road is heavily forested with military warning signs to **Keep Out**. Occasionally, an interesting plane would take off; next you would get a fighter jet. I'm amazed at how fast they move off the ground before disappearing into the sky.

My breakfast stop is in a small town called Mexico Beach, a slow-moving place compared to Panama Beach – no high-rise condos, just lots of very cool oceanfront bungalows and more great beaches. They call this area the Forgotten Coast, which will probably soon be rediscovered. Riding into town, I'm thinking about camarón (Spanish for *shrimp*) breakfast tacos. No such luck. I didn't see one Mexican restaurant, so I settled for a three-egg omelet, two large orange juices, and jam on toast. You can really work up an appetite when you're on the road!

My next stop is Port St. Joe, Home of the Florida Constitution. From there, the road takes me inland and I lose my beach scenery until I arrive in Apalachicola. Their town motto is "World's Best Oysters and Beaches." This is it! I'm having oysters for lunch! A local recommends Papa Joe's Oysters Bar and Grill. He wasn't wrong. The oysters were out of this world!

I'm watching James shuck my oysters. He tells me he has been doing this for sixty years. He has the hands of a bricklayer. I ask him where the oysters are from, and with a smile, he looks up and says, "They are from Colorado." If you haven't heard of Rocky Mountain Oysters, go look it up on Google.

The lady serving me is James's wife, and they have been married for fifty years. He tells more stories. He tells one story about a cyclist that he put up for the night. He used to keep in touch but has not heard from him in years. His wife starts chatting over the bar with another lady right next to me about the town gossip, medical stuff, and more stories. I contribute to their conversations now and then while enjoying the oysters.

On the wall behind the bar is a picture of Papa Joe on his boat. It's an old wooden cruiser, probably from the sixties. I can smell that boat – the damp wood and diesel fuel floating around in the bilge. James points to a guy in the restaurant and says, "That's Papa Joe's son, who now runs the place." When I came into the restaurant, a younger guy held open the door so I could bring in my bike and keep an eye on it. That younger guy is Papa Joe's grandson.

I pay my bill, but before I leave, I put my hand out to thank James for the stories and the excellent dozen and a half oysters I just polished off. He grabs my hand with a firm grip. He looks at me and says something like, "You be safe out there. Stop back sometime!" These words go straight over my head, but in his eyes, I can see his whole life. I see every story he told me and more about him, right there.

Twenty-five miles more takes me back across the water over long bridges that connect a bunch of small islands. I'm starting to see road signs warning about bears. That's a little troubling. Hopefully, the bears go after the crazy dogs!

Regarding the Florida Iron Man event this weekend, I'd like to give a shout out to Sara, my personal nutritionist for many years, and Ron, my personal trainer.

Tomorrow will be the end of the scenic beach towns along the Gulf of Mexico as I will be making my way east. I'm hoping to make it into Perry Thursday night.

Stats for the Day:

Distance travelled – 93.4 miles/150 kilometers
Average speed – 13.9 mph/22 kph
Time – 6 hours 40 minutes
Calories burned – 6,004

The Route:

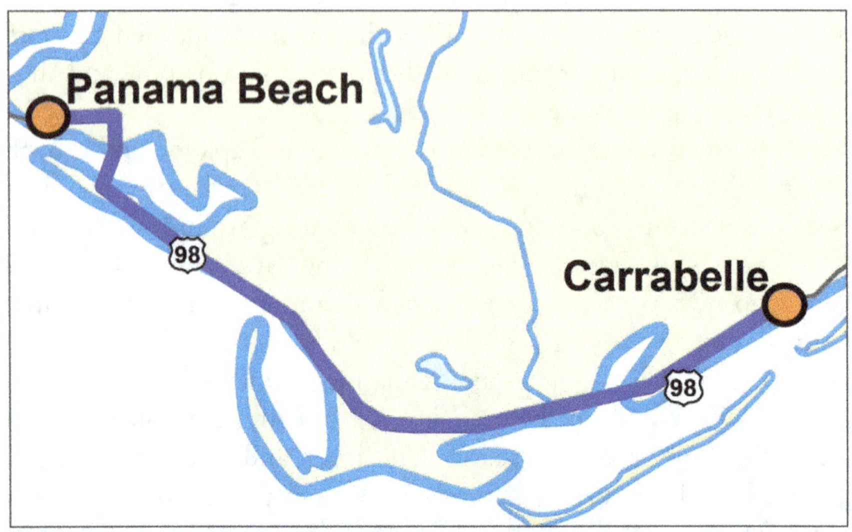

From Panama Beach to Carrabelle, Florida.

Pictures of the Day:

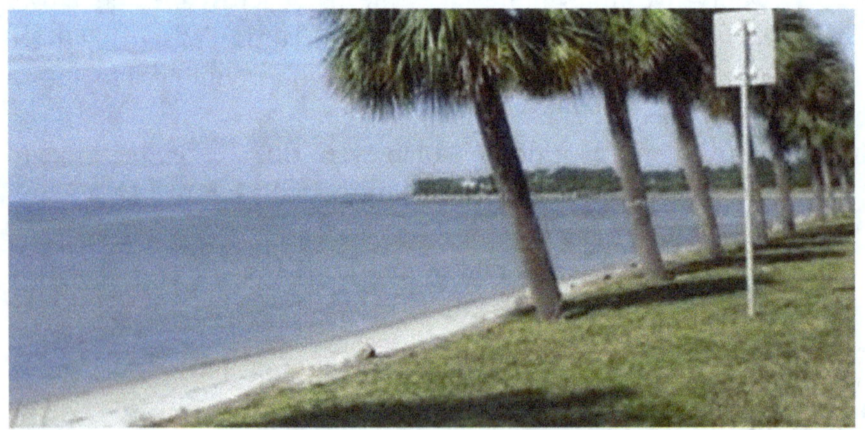

Some beach . . . somewhere.

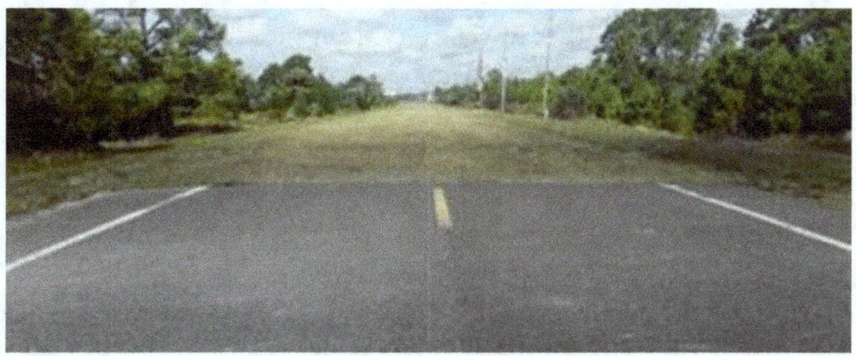

The end of the road literally.

Day 5: Thursday, November 5, 2015

Carrabelle to Perry, Florida – 86 miles/137 kilometers

Everything is good. It's the end of day five with 506 miles completed and 175 miles to go.

Its humid tonight in Perry, Florida. The fan turns slowly above me while I sit here trying to sew a few paragraphs together about today.

The day started early under gray skies, low ceiling, and a cool headwind. The road hugs the coast until I head north over Ochlockonee Bay. The clouds are getting lower and I can see the rain coming across the bay. Here we go again!

I'm really getting concerned about the bears. The girl serving breakfast this morning said that a couple of people got mauled over the summer. Usually the bears are going for garbage cans or react if they are startled. I asked, "What night is garbage night?" A little further down the road in a park, there's a bin on its side with garbage everywhere. Further on down the road there are residential garbage cans waiting for collection.

Both sides of the road are now tropical forest with slim, tall trees and ferns growing below. Now and then, I'd hear movement on the side of the road and quickly look to see a flock of doves. Up ahead I see three black images moving on the side of the road. I'm cautious as I close in. There are three little black pigs and they start to run, bumping into each other to get away from me. Not sure if they are wild pigs, but they would make good bacon by the look of them.

I have to stop and take a break. There's a small sandy road off to the side, and I head down about fifty yards to get away from the main road. I'm already concerned about bears, and here is a sign posted right in front of me about bears (see below). Okay. Okay. I know about the bears, but I need to take a break.

The rain eventually comes in, but it's only a light shower that lasts for a couple of hours. It's refreshing and helps to cool me down. The temperate is about 80°F (25°C) and very humid.

Coming into Perry, there is another great seafood eatery, Deal's Place. But it's too early for me to eat so I continue on. I'm now thinking about accommodations for tonight, when out of the corner of my eye I see a large brown dog heading for me at full speed. The dog has a collar and a long rope attached. The hair on my body stands on end as I launch into a full sprint. He misses me and ends up sliding halfway across the road trying to get traction to chase me. A large truck is not far behind me so the dog gives up. That is another victory for me – Dogs 0 versus Shane 1,550 (seems like that number anyway).

On the way back from dinner, there are a couple of blokes sitting on their Harleys outside their room enjoying some beers. I say, "G'day, mates," and they instantly offer me a cold beer. These couple of words with the right accent at the right time and place are as good as cash. After a couple more beers, we have completely covered the major topics of motorcycles and touring. Both Mark and Wesley live close to Daytona Beach and are heading to Apalachicola for the weekend seafood festival. And yes, they will call into Papa Joe's for some of those oysters and stories.

Tomorrow is a century ride (or 100 miles) to Gainesville, Florida.

Stats for the Day:

Distance travelled – 86 miles/138.4 kilometers
Average speed – 14.9 mph/24 kph
Time – 5 hours 46 minutes
Calories burned – 5,713

The Route:

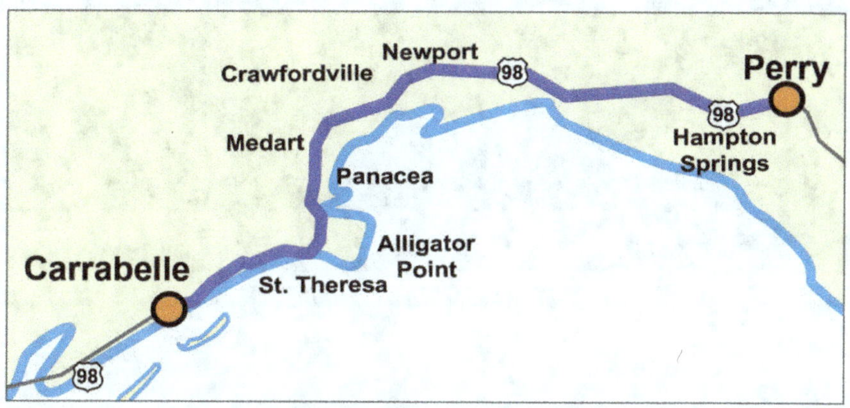

From Carrabelle to Perry, Florida.

Pictures of the Day:

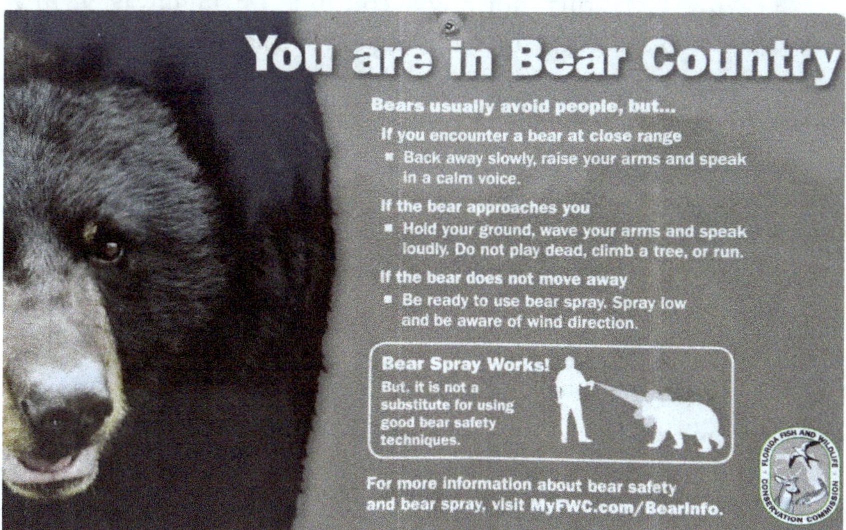

Bear spray looks easy enough to use.

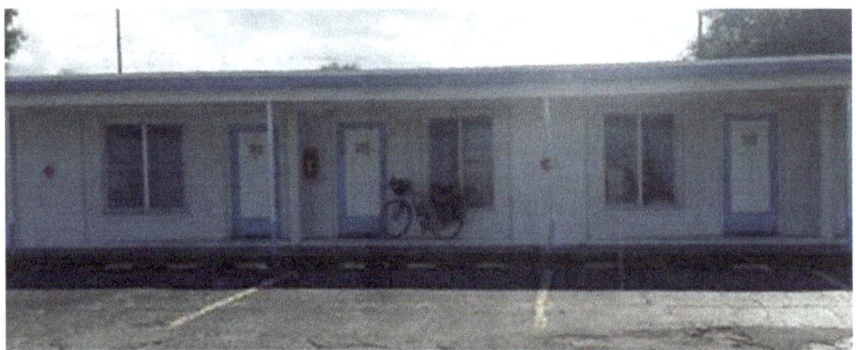

The Perry "Ritz-Carlton."

Day 6: Friday, November 6, 2015

Perry to Gainesville, Florida – 96 miles/154 kilometers

Leaving Perry this morning I continue on Highway 98. I've been on this black strip since leaving Pensacola. The morning was heavy with humidity which they say is unusual weather for this time of year. This area normally gets frost in the morning by now. The balmy weather allows me to dress light, so no switching out gloves and jackets during the morning.

I had breakfast this morning at the Cypress Creek Café in Cross City where we got into a detailed conversation about bears and safety. One of the girls said that bears can't run downhill, and that's a good way to get away from them. But there are no hills in Florida, from what I have seen anyway. Another suggested the best protection, other than a gun, is to bring a buddy that is slower than you. This apparently increases your survival rate from 50 percent to 87 percent, depending on how slow your mate is.

The café is run by a family, and young Toby is sitting at the bar next to me asking a bunch of questions about my ride. His grandmother is at the cash register and asks Toby why he isn't in school. He gives her some answer that seems to satisfy the question. I pay the bill, bid everyone a great day, then head out the door. As I'm unlocking my bike, I hear, "Come back, Shane!" Toby and grandma are now out the front of the restaurant and giving me directions to the Florida Bicycle Trail.

This trail is about 35 miles long. It's an old train route that is now a nice bike path, and since there are no trucks or cars, I can relax a little. The next thing I see is a snake about two feet long going across the path! I just miss running over its tail with my front wheel. That's it? A two-foot-long snake? In the southwestern deserts that would be a five- to six-foot rattlesnake!

I'm clipping along the path about 17 mph, head down and concentrating on the next twenty to thirty feet of pathway when *boom* – another snake! This one is black and about five feet long. I see him at the last minute and he just misses going under my back wheel.

As the day rolls on, I like to try and get a little bicycle yoga in, just to loosen everything up. I do a couple of child poses, some downward dogs (which are dangerous on a bike), followed by a few sun salutations. Yeah, that should do it for today.

After Trenton it's smooth sailing into Newberry on the outskirts of Gainesville with the usual city traffic. I've almost got the day done when I spot a large white cooler (known as an Esky in Australia) on the patio of a house, and in large blue hand-painted letters, it says "DAVE'S" on the side. I'm thinking this guy is pretty smart. At a party, everyone knows that it's Dave's cooler. No one is going to take it because it's *Dave's*. People say, "Oh yeah, that's *Dave's* cooler, but we have never met him." The cooler has taken on its own personality, setting it apart from the other coolers. Everywhere it goes, it stands out as **DAVE'S**. Even I know it's ***Dave's*** cooler. Is that a new business opportunity – personalizing coolers?

Tomorrow is my final day of this great adventure with 87 miles to the finish. I really can't believe it's coming to an end after five years. If I stacked the days back to back, it has taken thirty-two riding days to complete 2,820 miles across the southern United States, crossing through three different time zones and eight beautiful states. I've seen the most picture perfect landscapes, greeted the sunrise every day, and met a host of interesting characters who were always eager to help me or just have a yarn. It has been a gratifying and wonderful experience, for which I am grateful.

Tonight I'm in Gainesville, Florida, and there is a college football game being played. Every man and his dog are here. This has caused a spike in the low budget hotel rates.

Usually the last day is easy because your mind and body know it's done. I'm looking forward to seeing the Atlantic Ocean!

Stats for the Day:

Distance travelled – 96 miles/155.5 kilometers
Average speed – 14.9 mph/24 kph
Time – 6 hours 25 minutes
Calories burned – 6,360

The Route:

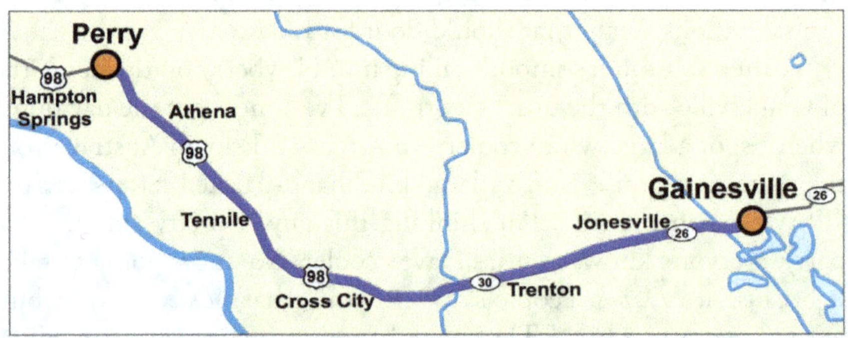

From Perry to Gainesville, Florida.

Pictures of the Day:

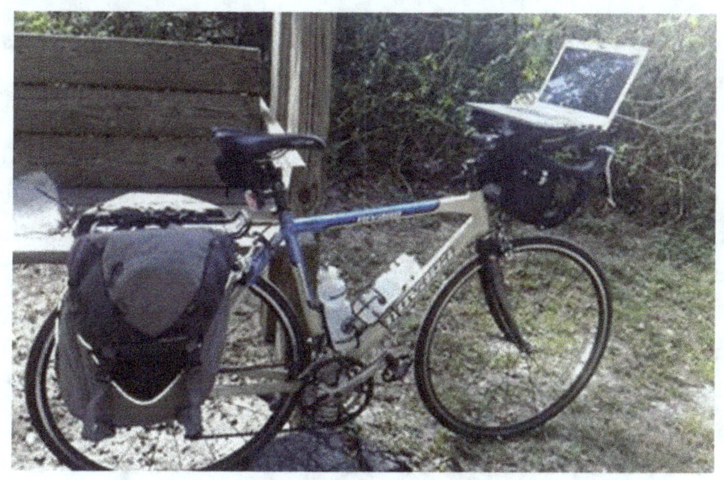

Is this at all possible? No.

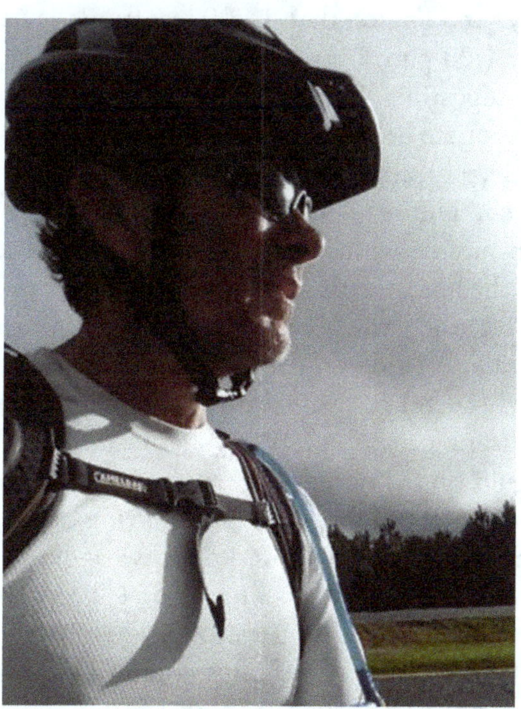

The rider writer. Say that quickly three times.

Day 7: Saturday, November 7, 2015

Gainesville to St. Augustine Beach, Florida – 84 miles/127 kilometers

It's an early start today. I'm excited to see the Atlantic Ocean and spend the weekend in St. Augustine, Florida, with Sara. I'm already thinking about next week and a business conference in Orlando that I'll be attending. Forget that. Enjoy the last day. This is it!

The weather is warm for November and it's sunny and humid. I'm happy not to be riding this in the summer. There's not much elevation change in Florida, maybe a couple of hundred feet if that. I passed through a number of small towns, taking Highway 26 south of Santa Fe Lake to Putnam Hall, then on to Route 100 to the Saint John's River and the small town of Palatka. I'm now on Route 207 to 206, which is a straight shot to Crescent Beach. Finally, I cross the Matanzas River and I'm less than 1,200 feet from the Atlantic Ocean.

At about 1:00 p.m. I arrive at Crescent Beach, about 11 miles south of St. Augustine. There's a final sand dune with a wooden walkway to negotiate before getting to see the ocean.

I take a deep breath of fresh, sweet, salty air as I look out across this wide beach. The sea is calm with only a small wave here and there that runs up the white sand. The beach looks endless in either direction and the blue ocean is a magnificent sight. It's so blue that it is difficult to see where the ocean ends and the sky begins.

It's low tide so I ride on the hard sand at the water's edge. I'm feeling relieved. There's no more traffic, no endless white line or crazy dogs, no trucks, no cars, no bears, no snakes, and best of all, there is no pain. Seagulls on the water's edge just stare as I ride by.

There are a few people swimming, playing on the water's edge, or just getting some sun. No one knows what has just happened. Some stop and watch as I cycle along. I'm feeling a sense of achievement and very thankful as my tires touch the water of the Atlantic Ocean. My doubts and fears that this couldn't be accomplished are gone. What started as a thought is now a reality – bicycling from a beach in San Diego on the Pacific Ocean across the southern United

States of America – 2,820 miles (4,538 kilometers) to the Atlantic Ocean!

I spend the next six miles riding on the hard sand at the water's edge at a slow pace. I'm about six miles from my hotel just south of St. Augustine.

I start to relive every day of this adventure, thinking back to when Sara dropped me off at the Phoenix airport for the first stage, my concerns about doing this solo, my thoughts walking back up Ocean Beach in California after dipping my rear wheel in the Pacific Ocean, then commencing in the San Diego morning traffic. These concerns diminished, and turned into confidence with each mile I rode and as each stage was completed. I knew things had changed once I crossed the mountains and survived the lonely stretches of west Texas. I learned a little bit more about myself and the reasons for taking this journey and how that changed along the way. It wasn't only about why to ride but about the changes in life over five years. This was an adventure combining a project, a goal, my family, my friends, my business, and life in general.

St. Augustine is the oldest, continuously occupied European-established settlement in the United State founded in 1565 by the Spanish. The city served as the capital of Spanish Florida for over two hundred years, and became the capital of British East Florida when the territory briefly changed hands between Spain and Britain. Spain ceded Florida to the United States in 1819. The town became known for pirates, and today is a famous tourist spot for visitors wanting to experience the older times. It's worth a look, with lots of history and old buildings that are now bars and restaurants.

I wonder if the people who discovered St. Augustine had the same feeling of fulfillment after they crossed the Atlantic Ocean centuries ago. Maybe similar to all the people who I met along the way, their lives were filled with amazing stories.

The one thing I didn't expect or anticipate starting out on this adventure was how other people enjoy the complete experience from my daily emails. Their feedback was very positive. This only made the journey more fun, and it was *truly* appreciated. Some people dusted off their old bikes and started riding, others decided it was time to join, or go back to the gym.

People ask me, "What were the biggest takeaways from this adventure?"

I would have to say it would be *pain, persistence, and people*. I believe that these are challenges we all face in our daily lives, whether on a bicycle or just living. While riding, my mind would wander to different subjects, like going up a steep hill in the heat of the day or a strong, never-ceasing headwind. For this I would feel the *pain* of my legs or the weight of my body on the saddle. Then came *persistence* to just keep going – you are almost there! I started thinking about *people,* the unique struggles they may be having in their life – the good and the bad, the lucky and the unlucky. These were the topics that were thought about every day of my ride. Sometimes though, going down a nice hill, there would be no pain and usually the most incredible views wide open before me. The beauty of it all could be overwhelming.

This adventure has been a true sense of achievement for me and an experience of a lifetime. I hope my story motivates others to follow their dreams and fulfill their own adventures. You never know whom you will inspire on your adventure while finding out about yourself along the way!

Stats for the Day:

Distance travelled – 84 miles/135 kilometers
Average speed – 14.9 mph/23 kph
Time – 5 hours 38 minutes
Calories burned – 5,518

The Route:

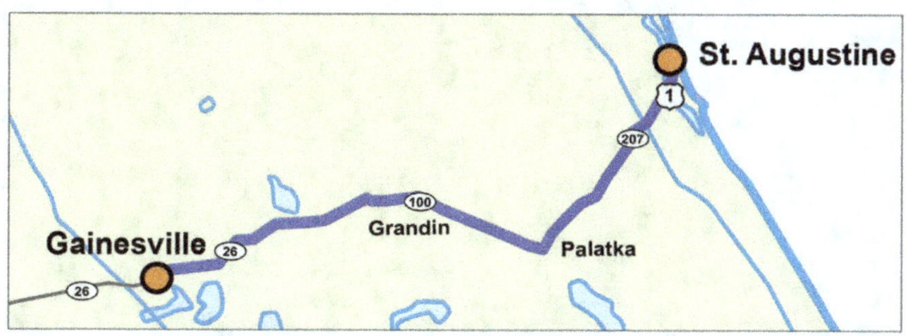

From Gainesville to St. Augustine Beach, Florida.

Picture of the Day:

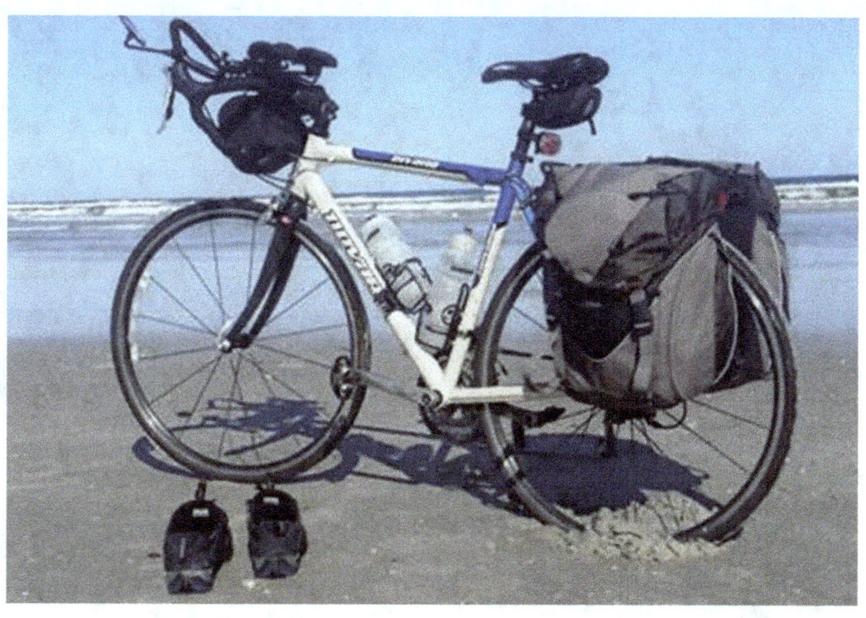

T H E   E N D

THE FINAL CHAPTER

You just can't finish an adventure like this without giving credit all the people that helped make this possible and inspire me along the way.

Stage 1 – San Diego to Phoenix

- *Got your email on the ride . . . good work! I used to ride religiously, and your email got me back in the saddle!*
- *I saw the email, that bike ride looked like an amazing experience . . . I'm a little jealous!*
- *Hi Shane Congratulations for having made your trip. It was a "quirk of fate" that we met you at Mission Trails Regional Park. I am so glad we did. We are volunteers there and have been for 5 years. However, we only work there 2 days a month, for 4 hours. So the chance of running into you were rather remote, to say the least. Really, really glad we did! I wish we had more time to see what you were doing. As it was we had no idea, as we got busy with what we were supposed to be doing. As it developed we were most impressed and greatly followed every aspect of it. I was concerned about your well being on highway 60 'to when I could not pick up your daily briefing. That is why I contacted a friend of yours, however, he eased my mind. What concerned me, was, a near tragedy for my wife, on that highway. Ruth, who you met, my wife of 61 years, and I used to, for many years ride motorcycles. Finally quit at age 75 out of common sense I guess. Anyway, we were on our Honda Gold wing one time in June, headed for the Grand Canyon. About 8 miles or so west of the intersection at Hope, where of*

course you took photo, we were cruising along, Ruth tapped me on the shoulder, I then pulled over. She was dizzy and felt bad. We removed her helmet, continued on so the wind would help her cool off. I told her there was a roadside store about 5-8 miles up the road. So we made it there and greatly concerned about heat stroke. We laid her out on picnic table in the shade of tree behind store at Hope (Quite likely you may have sat at same tree in the shade) I bathed her face with water etc and she started to recover. After several hours she seemed to be OK. Operators of the store offered to call ambulance, but I thought we had just barely solved our problem. We later aborted our Grand Canyon plans and went to Prescott and later Colorado River. At the store, she weakly asked for potato chips be because of desire for salt. SO, you can see why I was concerned about you! Anyway, very glad to have made your brief acquaintance. If out this was contact us! For the last 5 years we have lived in an up-scale mobile home park in Santee. We left our 10 acre ranch in the mountains after 36 years to be closer to medical facilities. We lived 30 miles north of Julian at same elevation. For many years I was a resident deputy sheriff there (for San Diego County) and did that all over the desert and mountains.

- *From Richard the other Aussie in the Desert: Well done. I sometimes think that is what life's about: setting goals and achieving them. I have a sneaky feeling I have bought some of your software (ROI rings a bell) a few years back when I was a CIO. I will check. With luck I will finish in San Diego tomorrow.*
- *From Tony the www.theworldjog.com: Just finishing breakfast in Cactus. They say they know you and your wife here! Thanks for the update I enjoyed it. Also for the brekkie yesterday :) And your help/advice re: I 10. I stopped at the highway patrol office in Welden and got permission, so will see how that goes, California by tomorrow night :)*
- *Thinking about you today. Hope you're well and strong. Weather looks good and hope the wind is at your back.*
- *Good Luck Mate, my thoughts and prayers are with you!*
- *I believe in you & I guess Sunscreen is Futile . . . Go Shane Go!*

Stage2 – Phoenix to El Paso

- *Congratulations on completing the recent leg of your bike adventure. That was a bummer with all of the flats. Some very late [advice] regarding the fine wire flats. I found that it was easy to locate the area of the flat because the wire was sticking out of the tire. So, rather than remove the wheel I would let it attached to the bike and release the tire from the rim in the area of the flat just enough to get the tube out to repair. Also, since the puncture is so small a glueless patch worked very well. Very important; remove the wire before replacing the tube into the tire and the tire onto the rim. Inflate and you are on your way. Could take less than 5 minutes for the entire operation. This is good if you have more interstate on your next leg. As you may already know, San Antonio is a great destination and the ride gets much more interesting from there on.*

- *That took you 5 days to make it on your bicycle? I could of made it in 1 1/2 days on my motorcycle.*

- *Very impressed with your performance; thank you for these reports and photos of your ride. I feel you had good times during your trip. Your example is inspiring, and I had the idea of trying to do a long ride this summer too; if this comes to completion, I would like to try riding from Paris to Tulle the city where my father leaves and where I will go on holidays; it's about 470 km depending on the road; for now it's just an idea, I need to get prepared and organized. Anyway, I will follow on riding during the weekend and get prepared for joining you on one of your next leg . . .*

- *Your emails and photos were really interesting. You have to know what you are doing out there on the road, especially repairing tires. It's hard to believe you can repair that many tires and still bike 124 miles in 10 hours. I forward your emails to Bill because he can't wait to check out the daily progress. It's inspiring for him and amazing to me.*

- *When are you planning to take on the 600 miles from El Paso to San Antonio? I'll bet it is hot riding right now. Thanks for the updates and we are happy you met the goals you set these bike trips you take are amazing man!! What possesses you to do this . . . ? Did you do make these long trips before you came to the US? Really impressive. Let's tap a few at your keg and talk about this soon . . .*

- *Wow – I know airfare is expensive these days from Phoenix to El Paso when traveling for business . . . Shane, absolutely amazed that you can ride this far –be safe and thanks again for your invaluable support.*

- *From Rick the cross country elliptical rider: I am safe and comfortable here in Superior, AZ. Thought I would stay at the local Fire Department but did not work out and staying in a motel instead. Thursday was supposed to be an easy 20 mile day, which turned into a tough 61 miler instead. Looks like you had quite a long one today. 50 miles to El Paso will be a snap. Have a safe flight home.*

- *Wow! Don't know how you do it mate, but keep it up. [It's] been great reading your daily updates . . . good job!!*

- *Shane! What a day! And what an adventure! I'll drink a cold one for you, too*

- *I can't believe the day you have had. UGH All those flats. You actually had that many tubes or you had to repair the same one or two several times? That I10 sounds like a nightmare. I do hope your last leg is filled with a wind at your back, good weather and no trucks or snakes.*

- *My idol, very impress, I will drink a beer for your hard effort today, keep up the great work.*

- *Shane, sounds like a very lonely road you were on. Did you feel anxious/vulnerable being so isolated like that? Looking forward to the next two days!*

- *Wow What a day. Snakes and a strange girl. The sunset pic is great. All these miles of nothing does leave one a bit exposed. Onward to another leg tomorrow. Be safe.*

- *How fantastic and exciting it must be to be on the road again. Keep the updates coming. The family is also all very interested to hear how you're getting along. Have a[n] extra safe trip, enjoy your journey.*

- *Great to receive on-line news of your trip. I wish you all the best for this new challenge, and I'm pretty sure you're enjoying yourself along the road. On my side I'm still keeping practicing and experiencing with sport; beginning of May I tried something new: 1 week of diet + trekking in the south of France; this was a great experience, despite only surviving on water, tea and clear soup we managed to walk 4 to 5 hours every day. Over the weekend I'm also trying to keep on cycling in the south of Paris, now my average trip is 80 km within 3 hours . . . maybe I'll be ready for joining you next year.*

- *Good on you mate. I'm impressed and will continue to follow your progress.*

- *That is fantastic, well done. Please keep sending updates. I am really jealous.*

- *That is great! Uphill and hot are not my strengthens.*

- *Good going, Shane! I think you got the hardest part out of the way!*

- *Happy to hear the first day was a success and you're smiling over at least one pint:) I greatly appreciate your keeping me on the mailing list as I look forward to doing this ride with you day by day. Watch out for the snakes.*

- *Shane. I just registered for the "Tour de Cure" (Diabetes) . . . 80 miles, falls right in my training plan. March 24. You might be on the road then; don't recall your dates. Keep it in mind.*

Stage 3 – El Paso to San Antonio

- *I am loving your trip journals! You are a great writer and perhaps a book about your experience may be in your future. We are thinking of you and pulling for you while you travel on your bike.*

- *Great Job Mate . . . I love all the great stories. Keep em coming. Once you get along the water it should be beautiful.*

- *Ride sounds great, appreciate the smooth pavement! The county chip seal folks are using aggregate the size of bowling balls in Salt Lake*
- *Just a note to let you know we're with you mate, enjoying your narrative as you proceed on your adventure*
- *Glad you decided to book ahead, think you should have a teaser for you for the approaching dogs, wildlife and stranger thou!*
- *I'm so jealous. If I come to work for you can I do this while on the job too?*
- *Shane keep up the awesome job you are an inspiration to many fulfilling your dream.*
- *Shane – enjoyed reading about your ride. Pretty sure that's a Plymouth Road Runner. Looks like it may have been modified (hood). Enjoy the journey!*
- *I think your armadillo is not just resting. Don't think they sleep on their backs. The car may be a 60s vintage Dodge Charger--from the "muscle car" era.*
- *Thanks mate for the update, your detailed email makes me feel like i am on the road with you . . . sooo cool.*
- *Shane, thanks for the update. I'm still riding, but still only dreaming of making the trip. Wow! 700 miles in 7 days. That's cookin', man! I'll follow you the whole way. Godspeed!*

Stage 4 – San Antonio to New Orleans

- *Excellent! I was honored to be a part of your trek. My boss Lisa actually saw your email and mentioned on my RAP.*
- *What you have done on the bike ride(s) is truly fantastic and you should be very proud of it.*
- *Congratulations on completing the latest leg of your trans-America challenge.*
- *I have to say I've thoroughly enjoyed reading your daily blogs, I think you have a real talent for it. I just imagine the looks on the faces of the locals when the alien from Oz lands in their*

isolated communities! You read very much like a Bill Bryson novel – succinct and witty observational humor.

- *You made it . . . awesome effort again! We are so proud of you. Your journey has inspired all of us here*
- *Very, VERY cool Shane. I've have read everyday's journal of your trip and really think you might have a future in travel blogs or cultural best sellers!*
- *Well done on the ride mate, and a very entertaining journey log so far, dare I say, ripe for a book and mini-series after you make it to the east coast. I have already shared some of your antics with the family (although that's nothing new),*
- *Really . . . swap people. Stef loves reading your updates and I often hear her laughing out loud.*
- *Great reading. I would love to do the same. Very motivating.*
- *I got to tell ya – you're a great writer. Entertaining, to the point, and we can all picture being there as you're describing things. Here in Pittsburgh, there are tons of cyclists and half of my office cycle to work each day. I've been forwarding your adventures to them each morning as they are really interested and we're having a great laugh together. Keep taking good care of yourself as you come to the close of this ride, and thanks for providing some great stories this week for all of us.*
- *I must say you are incredible, an amazing inspiration and motivation for me to get on the bike for real.*
- *Great reading your daily blog! I need to get out there and join you!*
- *I read out the emails and we just love hearing every day!!!*
- *This is awesome Shane! Just incredible. And getting to throw in a little business too. A bonus of sorts.*
- *It sounds like you are having quite an adventure. Thanks for sharing with those of us too lazy or old to do something like what you're doing. Your trip has made for enjoyable reading.*
- *Your excellent descriptions are making my mouth water for a ride of my own---only on my "bike" and on my terms. I have ridden that area (generally) some years back, but of course did not get the flavor of the areas like you have. But you have*

whetted my appetite for a trip along the Gulf Coast. My problem will be to slow down enough to "smell the roses" and savor the sights and the people. Your way is better in that sense, and I envy your fortitude and focus. Great trip, and thanks again for the running commentaries.

- *I love reading your daily updates! I seriously cannot wait for each one to Come!!! Great job!*

- *Sounds awesome. Extremely jealous of your adventure and always seem to find a way to incorporate business! Wishing you a safe rest of the trip and wanted to let you know that I really enjoy and look forward to your E-mails every day. These are going to make for a great book one day.*

- *I'm living vicariously through your messages and may get the courage to get off my couch because of you. I can reflect on times in my life when I felt strong and resilient. Whether that was through consistent exercise or simply by virtue of spending quality time with my kids. The latter is clearly a motivating piece of my life.*

- *Shane, you are making me want to go on an adventure!*

- *Fantastic! Didn't realize you were such a great writer as well as rider! Thanks for the wonderful vicarious escape.*

- *An amazing trip it is! I'm feeling jealous about your experience right now, me being stuck here working on the computer and having left the summer season with not enough biking as I was [busy] building this new life here in south of France (well, this is bad for good certainly) . . . I'll have my revenge one day ;-)*

- *So good again to have another update! Wow! What a great day . . . (this morning though) Don't even say about "why, crazy or silly"! It's just so awesome what you're doing! We have all just been sitting down stairs around in the camp chairs, and I read out your daily blog! It's so cool! We hang on your every word!!! And the Glen Campbell Galveston song last night was good! . . . As you said we turned up loud . . . Keep it coming and safe trip.*

- *Great reading you better start a book when you finish the last leg I'm sure people would love to read it. We have really been enjoying the details, looking at the map it's a shame you couldn't have gone straight ahead when you left this morning, but I guess that's a no go area or you would have! So is tonight in a motel or in a tent? Bet the shrimp was great not too keen on the cockys though. And luckily you didn't end up trapped in a cool room . . . stay safe . . .*

- *My husband is getting into your trip. Your adventures are wonderful escapes and my "behind" aches every time I read them. I have only ridden 100 miles once in my life. That was once enough.*

- *What a terrific story's! Your ride just has to make all of us couch potatoes green with envy. You're quite obviously having a wonderful time, and meeting some "salt of the earth" people.*

- *Great blog Shane — following your progress with great interest — your writing has become more entertaining too — got that Aussie spirit in it*

- *Mate I think you missed your calling. You should have been a writer. Marilyn always gets a laugh out of your emails Be safe Shane . . . A few things come to mind . . . 1st I've tallied around 17,000 calories you've burned mate, that's incredible. [You're] gonna be one skinny bastard when your done On a serious side . . . [you're] an inspiration. I wasn't going to work out today, but with what you're doing, I'm going right now. Enjoy the coast brother and can't wait to hear your next recap.*

- *I am so enjoying your daily recaps. You have the ability with your choice of words that I am smelling and seeing what you are. I appreciate that my body is not taxed like yours! When you write your book, I will be first in line to buy and have a signed copy.*

- *I LOVE reading your e-mails and tracking your progress. You write so beautifully — great "voice" and very descriptive. We feel we are experiencing this with you — without the agony, of course. Although it must not be all agony for you — but a great sense of accomplishment every "step" of the way.*

- *A road trip on a pushy is the best way to truly experience a journey. Reading your touring cycling yarn has inspired me to start planning my next ride.*
- *Jolly good blogging! I am really enjoying reading it. Your narrative skill is excellent. Thanks for including me.*
- *Sounds great, would have loved to have followed along behind you! Did you take a picture of the guy in Pop`s can nearly imagine what he looks like . . .*

Stage 5 – New Orleans to St. Augustine

- *Awesome adventure, mate! Congratulations on the finish, and I really enjoyed your riding journal. We definitely are kindred spirits and are going to have to do a ride someday. I have done 2700km of my Cross-Canada . . . only 4800km more to go! Yes, the Cross-Canada route is the widest section of the North American continent. Someday . . . Anyway, I looked forward to your daily emails and I ALMOST felt like I was on the ride with you. Well done.*
- *Well done Shane. Thanks for sharing. Very inspirational*
- *Well Done! Great Effort! Was thinking of following in your tire tracks until you mentioned the snakes!!!*
- *CONGRATULATIONS MATE. You did it! That's a great achievement – very few people would tackle that trip solo – that makes you a true adventurer.*
- *Great job – it's been great following your adventure all these years. Congratulations on getting it all done.*
- *So proud to know you buddy, you have really inspired all of us.*
- *Congratulations my friend, that is an amazing accomplishment. Think of all the people and all the places you've seen that you probably would never have experienced if it wasn't for this journey. I also think about all the people you've touched, leaving them with your upbeat positive spirit. Great job!*
- *Congratulations! A truly remarkable achievement. You continue to be an inspiration for me . . . thank you.*

- *Congratulations. I know from my personal experiences what you have achieved. We enjoyed your daily updates very much, and we have the feeling that we know that part of the US somehow better now. Well done.*
- *Great job and what an adventure. I lived through you along your journey Shane. Thank you for taking the time to share with us.*
- *Thanks my friend! I truly miss you. I will spend the next bunch of catch vicariously living through your 2015 adventures!*
- *Congratulations Shane. In the words of Jack Gibson: you've played hard, done good. I've enjoyed reading about your trip not just this year, but right from San Diego. My 19 year old grand daughter was in the office in the past week and I showed her your emails. She said WOW!*
- *Congrats on a good job done! You've done a nice trip, and I like the way you write your story, you've got a good sense of entertaining us with what is characteristic of the day. Very inspiring. Cheers from sunny Montpellier . . .*
- *Congratulations Shane! I have really enjoyed traveling with you on your grand adventure.*
- *This has been a great accomplishment. One that very few people have done. Buddy, you are an Iron Man, in the truest sense of the word. You are also a pretty good story teller.*
- *Well done mate, great journey and a wonderful way to see & experience life. After reading your daily reports I feel I know more about the States or certain people and places you have encountered. I love the freedom n surprises around every corner with touring on a bike*
- *Your blog is great! I am enjoying it immensely.*
- *Shane, you not only are an adventurer, you have a keen eye for detail and a poet's way of expression*
- *Good stories! I read your travels out loud to my family. Thanks for sharing and be safe!*
- *I am really enjoying your updates and hope you are enjoying your ride. What a wonderful endeavor to do this for a week each year. Even though I'm enjoying my retirement I have to*

admit I feel somewhat guilty that I am not making better use of my time like you are. You are a true inspiration

- *Too cool my friend! Keep living the dream!!!*
- *Awesome to get to follow you on this journey (at least via email) . . . keep it going!!!*
- *GREAT READ! "If I was with you we would have stopped in Bayou La Batre" Travel Safe!*
- *Thanks so much for sharing your stories as you experience them. Keep the details coming*
- *Looking forward to following your great adventure.*
- *I love your updates. I do have to say I was blown away yesterday. When you said bike ride I assumed you meant motorcycle. Imagine my surprise when I received the day 1 update.*
- *You bring tears to my heart, the experience, the journey. Such a wonderful memory you have of biking across America. So admire what you have done and last leg of it.*
- *Wish I was there. Let me tell you, some days I just wanna run away from the whole life thingo, and if I did maybe I would bike . . . I certainly would get fit anyway.*
- *Absolutely incredible that you've seen so much of this country on 2 wheels. AMAZING!*
- *So you're going to finish. I'm insanely jealous. In my mind, I'm still going to follow your footsteps!*

ABOUT THE AUTHOR

Shane Hannan moved to the United States in 1997. He met his wife in Whistler, Canada on a snow skiing adventure. They have a son and a daughter. Shane is a true entrepreneur and loves meeting people as he travels for business. Since 2003 he has owned a software company in Scottsdale, Arizona developing software solutions that are marketed and sold through distribution partners worldwide. He enjoys the outdoors and the warm climate of the sonoran desert. Previously he lived in Seattle for 3 years and prior to that lived in Sydney, Australia, growing up on the beaches of Cronulla, in the Sutherland Shire.

www.ingramcontent.com/pod-product-compliance
Lightning Source LLC
Chambersburg PA
CBHW070121260726
48658CB00001B/209